Effective Management in Long-term Care Organisations

A Textbook for Students and New Care Managers

Effective Management in Long-term Care Organisations

A Textbook for Students and New Care Managers

Janet Scott, Anne Gill and Keith Crowhurst

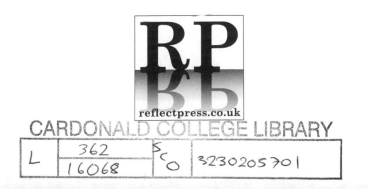

reflectpress.co.uk

First published in 2008

ISBN: 978 1 906052 02 7

British Library Cataloguing in Publication Data
A catalogue record for this book is available from the British Library

Production project management by Deer Park Productions, Tavistock, Devon
Typeset by Pantek Arts Ltd, Maidstone, Kent
Cover design by Oxmed
Printed and bound by Bell & Bain Ltd, Glasgow

www.reflectpress.co.uk

Published by Reflect Press Ltd
11 Attwyll Avenue
Exeter
Devon
EX2 5HN
UK
01392 204400

Contents

Introduction

This is a book for managers and future managers in long-term care settings including nursing homes, residential care homes and the variety of care settings in the community. It will enable readers to apply the theories and principles of management to the delivery of care and the management of staff. The book focuses on practice but includes a theoretical framework to enhance the reader's understanding of the practice. There is a balance between health and social care issues as the changes in the social care sector mean that many staff are now dealing with health issues.

WHY WE WROTE THE BOOK

When we were planning and validating a foundation degree in management for nursing home and social care managers we noticed that there are only a few books written specifically for people working in this area. There is also a shortage of management books suitable for newly appointed care managers. Most of the books we use as a basis for our teaching are heavily orientated towards management theory with few specifically written for health or social care managers at this level. There are also a large number of people taking NVQs (National Vocational Qualifications) Level 3 and 4 who are preparing for more senior positions in social care management. Many individuals taking management courses are preparing for careers in the social care sector and this book will be of help to them. The book also addresses the key skills framework and will be helpful to health service workers who need to achieve these competencies.

The book attempts to address a wide range of theory and practice and we have been careful to cover new developments such as reflection and clinical supervision, developing electronic records for the social care sector and new legislation including the National Standards Framework.

STANDARDS AND COMPETENCIES

The Care Standards Act (2000) introduced a new educational qualification for Managers of Nursing and Social Care Homes (The Registered Manager

Award or RMA). The new requirements for Registered Managers are outlined in Standard 31.2 of the Department of Health (2003, p. 38) report: *Care Homes for Older People National Minimum Standards*. The book also addresses the key skills that all health service personnel have to achieve to maintain their registration.

This book is therefore specifically focused on the National Occupational Standards for the Registered Manager Award, emphasising those standards relating to Managing Human Resources and Managing the Organisation. Specific standards are identified in relation to each chapter. The book will also provide information for those attempting to achieve the following competencies in the key skills framework at Level 4:

CD1   Communication: develop and maintain communication with people on complex matters, issues and ideas and/or in complex situations.

CD2   Personal and people development: develop oneself and others in areas of practice.

CD4   Service improvement: work in partnership with others to develop, take forward and evaluate direction, policies and strategies.

CD5   Quality: develop a culture that promotes equality and values diversity.

IK1   Information processing: develop and modify data and information management models and processes.

IK2   Information collection and analysis: plan, develop and evaluate methods and processes for gathering, analysing, interpreting and presenting data and information.

IK3   Knowledge and information resources: develop the acquisition, organisation, provision and use of knowledge and information.

G4   Financial management: plan, implement, monitor and review the acquisition, allocation and management of financial resources.

G6   People management: plan, develop, monitor and review the recruitment, deployment and management of people.

STRUCTURE

The book has been divided into three parts reflecting the book's main themes.

Part One: Managing People

This section deals with the many skills needed to manage people, starting with understanding the different roles utilised at work, managing oneself, and then building and managing a team, and concluding with a discussion of the principles of decision making and appraisal.

Part Two: Managing the Workplace

This section deals with managing the workplace. The starting point is how to recruit and select staff to meet the needs of the organisation and the information needed to achieve this. Workforce planning and skill mix follow with a detailed account of how to plan your workforce and ensure that the skill mix is right for you. The last two chapters in this part address the management of finances and resources to match the needs of the workplace and the workforce.

Part Three: Managing Change

This section deals with managing change, the starting point is sources of information and quality issues. Once problems are recognised change theory can be used appropriately through the use of skills of negotiation and managing conflict including complaints. Overall issues in the organisation can be tackled using strategic planning.

USING THIS BOOK

Case studies, reflection points and activities help you to interact with the text. The case studies are based on real-life situations and are intended to help you come to grips with the important management dilemmas that happen to us all. The reflection points focus on specific issues related to the topic and are also based on real-life experiences. Activities enable you to evaluate your own practice in relation to the topic. You are urged to answer the questions and complete the activities because, if you do, you will have the basis of a detailed management portfolio that will assist you in both your studies and your career as a manager. Please note that for all questions, reflections and activities you will be directed to relevant parts of the chapter and where appropriate, to further reading for information that will help you to answer them. However, you should also reflect on your experience of managing and/or being managed when responding to the questions asked.

AUTHOR BIOGRAPHIES

Dr Janet Scott SRN, SCM, BA (Hons), MSc, RNT, MA, PhD

Dr Janet Scott has experience of management in both health and education and has worked in Britain and New Zealand. At present she teaches health policy and health service management and participates in health service research. She is interested in the application of management principles to operational management in the health service including the implications of the changing roles of health workers. Janet was recently a Senior Lecturer at the University of Greenwich but is currently Director of Clinical Services Fatimah Memorial Hospital, Lahore, Pakistan.

Anne Gill SRN, DipN (Lond), Cert Ed, BSc (Hons), MSc

Anne Gill has a nursing background and has worked in Australia, Germany, Scotland and England. She has been involved in continuing professional development for health and social care workers since 1984. A more recent but related interest is in flexible learning for mature students utilising e.learning and blended learning. She is currently programme leader for a Foundation Degree in Care Management involving e.learning plus flexible attendance. She was also part of a team that developed a programme of clinical supervision workshops that is being used by NHS trusts throughout South-East England. Anne is currently a Senior Lecturer at the University of Greenwich.

Keith Crowhurst

Keith Crowhurst has had a career in nursing older people and he has worked in both the private and public sector. His current post is Home Manager for Sanctuary Care and Honorary Lecturer with the University of Greenwich. Keith has a keen interest in continuing education and his current role involves developing nursing units and their staff. Part of this role is to support care home managers through the use of tools such as reflective supervision and clinical governance.

ACKNOWLEDGEMENTS

We acknowledge each other's help in the writing of this book and the help and support of our publisher who has been very kind and patient with three new authors.

The publisher and authors would like to thank the following people/organisations for permission to reproduce their material in this book. Every attempt has been made to seek permission for copyright material used in this book. However, if we have inadvertently used copyright material without permission/acknowledgement we apologise and we will make the necessary correction at the first opportunity.

Figure 'Integrating performance management' from *Managing in the Public Sector* by B. Blundell and A. Murdock, Butterworth Heinemann, 1997, p. 96. Reprinted with permission of Elsevier Limited.

Figure 'Stages of group formation' found in *Organizational Behaviour* by Huczynski A. and Buchanan D., Prentice Hall 1991 based on *Group Organizational Studies: Stages of small group development revisted*, Tuckman, Bruce W. and Jensen Mary Ann C., 2, 419–427. Sage, Reproduced with permission of Pearson Education and Copyright Clearance Centre on behalf of Sage Publications Inc.

Figure 'The Functional Leadership Model' adapted from *Personnel and Human Resource Management* 5th edition by G.A. Cole, © Gerald Cole 2002. Reprinted with permission of Cengage Learning Services Limited.

Figures 'The decision model', 'A decision tree' and 'Appraisal Interview Styles' adapted from *Management Theory and Practice* 6th edition, by G. Cole 2004 Copyright © Gerald Cole 2004. Reprinted with permission of Cengage Learning Services Limited.

Figure 'Juran trilogy of total quality management' adapted from *Quality Improvement – Health Care Team Preparation Workbook*, Juran Institute 1993. Reprinted with permission.

Figure 'Resolving conflict through negotiation and mediations' from 'Management for Doctors: Conflict, power, negotiation' by L. Donaldson, *British Medical Journal* 310, 104–107, 1995. Reprinted with permission.

Figure 'Six key activities for successful implementation of change and figure 'The likelihood of long-term behaviour change' from *Managing Change and Making it Stick* by R. Plant, Fontana 1995.

Figure 'The learning curve' adapted from *Field Theory in Social Science* by Kurt Lewin, republished by APA (American Psychological Association books).

Figure 'Quality in action: the quality circle' from *Introducing Quality Assurance in the NHS* by T. Gould and H. Merrett, published by Palgrave Macmillan, 1992 pg 4. Reprinted with permission of Palgrave Macmillan.

Figure 'The clinical audit cycle' from *Making use of Clinical Audit: A Guide to Practice in the Health Professions* by M. Kogan and S. Redfern, published by Open University Press. Reprinted with the kind permission of Sally Redfern.

Figure 'Factors influencing roles in organisations' adapted from *The Social Psychology of Organizations* 2nd Edition, D. Katz and R.L. Kahn, John Wiley & Sons Ltd, 1978 pg 86, adapted version in 'Enactment in managerial jobs: A role analysis' by N. Fondas and R. Stewart, *Journal of Management Studies* V 31.1, Jan 1994, pp 83–103, Blackwells. Reprinted with permission of Wiley-Blackwell Publishing Ltd, and John Wiley & Sons Inc.

Figure 'Relationship Styles' from *Really Managing Health Care* 2nd edition by Valerie Iles. Reprinted with permission of the Open University Press Publishing Company.

Part One

Managing People

Chapter 1

Roles

INTRODUCTION

The topic of roles along with other topics in Part One will enable you to address National Occupational Standard A2 'Manage activities to meet requirements'. In this chapter you will:

- gain an understanding of the theory and definitions of roles;
- understand the implications of role uncertainty, conflict and ambiguity;
- reflect on the mutual role expectations of staff and managers;
- learn about managing role change and its consequences;
- understand the complexities of the manager's role and reflect on your own role within your organisation.

DEFINING ROLES

'A role in an organisation is normally considered to be a set of behaviours expected by others' (Buchanan and Huczynski, 2004). The concept of 'role' is used to understand the behaviour of people in organisations. A person may have a single role or may undertake many roles at the same time, as seen in Figure 1.

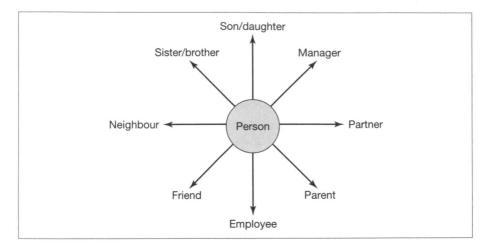

Figure 1 The roles people have in daily life

A role in an organisation refers to the point of contact between an individual and an organisation (Hales, 1986). Role attributes are what an organisation expects the employee or manager to be. Organisations can therefore be considered to be a collection of roles that act as the 'skeleton' that holds an organisation together.

ROLE UNCERTAINTY

An important function of role relationships is to reduce the areas of possible uncertainty to manageable proportions (Buchanan and Huczynski, 2004). This is important as, for example, managers' jobs can be loosely defined, are negotiable and can be influenced by the person holding the job as well as by the organisation and its resources. Uncertainty in a role can lead to insecurity and strain for both employees and managers. Organisations and the roles within them have become more complex due to the rapid pace of change (Handy, 1999) and this can increase role uncertainty. Insecurity can also be increased if there is uncertainty about how one's work will be evaluated (Handy, 1999): for example, there is no written description of the role. It is therefore important that both individuals and the organisation should have a clear idea of what is expected of each role. In formal organisations what a person should do when they play a specific role is usually written in a job description. Predetermined roles may be unexciting, but they do provide certainty (Handy, 1999). One of the strengths of formal organisations is that roles remain constant despite the turnover of staff in posts (Katz and Kahn, 1978). However, this can also be a weakness if the organisation changes so much that the prescribed roles are no longer relevant, which may then impede the progress of the organisation.

MANAGING ROLE EXPECTATIONS

The organisation's expectations of a particular role are normally communicated to the post holder using a job description. As can be seen in Figure 2, not only are job descriptions used in formal evaluations of behaviour (for example, appraisals) but they also influence and bring about conformity with the expectations of the role in question. This 'sent' role is the way organisations communicate with their members. However, expectations about roles also exist in people's minds and this can induce the required behaviour (Katz and Kahn, 1978). Problems can occur when the messages sent by the organisation about a role are distorted or misunderstood by the post holder because of their own perception of what the role should be. The 'received' role will therefore be subjective and depend on the personality, interests, values, motivation and perceptions of the post holder (Katz and Kahn, 1978). Expectations are often unplanned by organisations and may alter over time, as external pressures change (Flanagan and Spurgeon, 1996). Therefore, managing role expectations is a vital element in maintaining a role system within an organisation.

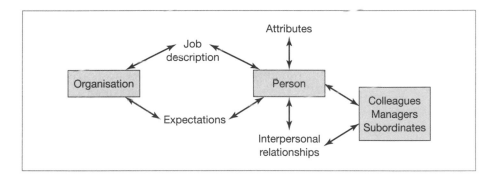

Figure 2 Factors influencing roles in organisations (adapted from The Katz and Khan 1978 Model)

Reflection

It was noticeable that when nurse education moved from hospitals and into higher education institutions as a result of Project 2000, the students had difficulty in being accepted by other registered nurses, as well as by patients, relatives and other qualified professionals. Part of the problem may have been the expectations that others had of their role. The students had received a different type of training, yet they were still expected to undertake the role of a traditional staff nurse. Neither their colleagues nor the organisations had changed their expectations of the role.

1. If you were managing an organisation in these circumstances what would you do to ensure the students' new role was understood and accepted? (See Managing Role Expectations.)

Role conflicts and ambiguity

Individuals will come to an organisation with expectations about the role that they are going to fulfil (Buchanan and Huczynski, 2004). Role conflict can occur if the organisation is not explicit, for example, in their job description as regards the scope of responsibility, participation in decision-making, limits of authority, company rules, job security and the way work is evaluated. This can lead to misunderstandings by all concerned. Misunderstandings can lead to ambiguity and lack of confidence on the part of the new employee or manager, as well as irritation and perhaps anger from other staff. Role problems can also cause deterioration in interpersonal relationships (Handy, 1999). The clarification of expectations has been shown to increase performance, and gives scope for the use of initiative and intelligence on the part of a manager (Buchanan and Boddy, 1992). Within organisations there are many groups who conceive their own norms of what is correct behaviour and they have expectations of what people in certain positions do (Schein, 1970). Every occupant of every position in a group is expected to carry out certain functions when one group interacts with another (Buchanan and Huczynski, 2004) and people respond to the expectations that others have of their role (Dopson and Stewart, 1993).

Reflection

It can be difficult for a Health Care Assistant who then goes on to train as a nurse to go back to the same part of an organisation after their training. There will be people working in that department who have expectations that the work relationships and friendships will remain as before, despite the HCA's change in qualification and role.

1. Reflect on your expectations of the role of a care assistant in your organisation. What exactly do you expect them to do?
2. Colleagues often feel that people 'change' when promoted. What do you think? Is it simply the change in role or do colleagues reactions also change? (See Managing Role Expectations and Changing Staff Roles.)

Overcoming role ambiguity

One way of overcoming role ambiguity is to provide feedback as a measure of performance (Handy, 1999). This is particularly relevant in times of change as it can clarify the 'unspoken' expectations of their role for role holders. It can also eliminate any confusion that can arise as to how performance will be measured. Feedback should be constructive, and positive as well as negative feedback should be given. Within the health service positive feedback has always been a problem, and to such an extent that many managers consider the lack of negative feedback as positive feedback.

It is particularly important to provide feedback after a reorganisation of the management structure in an organisation. Expectations of roles may have changed as a result and these expectations need to be made explicit. Feedback needs to be provided, both within and outside of an appraisal system. It is difficult for employees to achieve exactly what is required without constructive feedback (Iles, 1997). Many appraisal systems only provide feedback at specific intervals such as, for example, annually or six monthly. If there is uncertainty, or problems with performance, feedback should be provided more regularly to enable post holders to change their performance and reduce the stress which can be caused by role ambiguity.

Reflection

I had been in a manager's post for 18 months when I suddenly received negative feedback. I was told that I had not been performing well since I had come into the post. I had thought I had been performing well as I had not received any negative feedback. The fact that I had not received positive feedback was not unusual for the organisation that I worked in and I had received some performance-related pay. Part of the difficulty was as a result of expectations. The job was a new post and my immediate manager's expectations of my role differed from mine. However, he had not made his expectations explicit and he had not provided me with any specific feedback over the period.

1. How do you provide feedback in your organisation? (See Managing Role Expectations.)
2. What are your expectations of the role of your manager? Has your manager made their role explicit to you? (See Managing Role Expectations and Managers' Roles in an Organisation.)

Key Learning Points

Role conflict and ambiguity occur when there is uncertainty about:

- How a role holder's work is evaluated;
- Their scope for advancement;
- Their scope for responsibility;
- Others' expectations of their performance.

Changing staff roles

Managers may well expect employees to change their roles in reaction to a new regime. They may ask role holders to take more or less responsibility. Also, if a new manager is employed, employees may take the opportunity to attempt to change their own role, to expand their role or to discard responsibilities they dislike. This negotiation process is interactive and the manager must be aware of the possible traps. They should neither raise expectations unrealistically nor suppress what may be creative reactions to the new situation. A positive approach would be to review organisational goals and targets with the team and individuals, and to allocate roles and responsibilities in relation to abilities, potential and the needs of the organisation.

MANAGERS' ROLES IN AN ORGANISATION

Job descriptions

Job descriptions at middle management level, while listing the formal aspects of the job, rarely say anything about the informal, more subtle, unspoken expectations (Katz and Kahn, 1978). Only by comparing the manager's own perceptions of what their job is with their formal job description can you really distinguish between the formal and informal aspects of their work (Hales, 1986).

Negotiating job content

Managers can influence their job descriptions and this often makes it more likely that they will succeed. Managers can negotiate the content of their role as part of the job they do by, perhaps, concentrating on what they do best and at the same time discarding the parts of their role that they dislike by delegation. Of course, this is more likely to happen when a job is less formally defined and the organisation encourages a culture of collaboration and team work. It is expected that some changes will occur whenever a new manager comes into post. In fact, the more proactive the manager is in deliberately using opportunities to change employees' expectations of both their role and the manager's role, the more likely they are to be successful. In addition, the new manager must ensure that their own line manager is aware of how they intend to fulfil the role. Managers need to be aware that: 'self created expectations are potentially more easily fulfilled, and they can fill a void created by for example, an organization's mission or resource uncertainty, its rapid growth, conflict among role senders or other factors ...' (Fondas and Stewart, 1994, p. 98).

> **Key Learning Points**
>
> Roles in an organisation can be:
>
> - Prescriptive – as shown on a job description;
> - Evaluated – in an appraisal;
> - Descriptive – based on the actual duties performed;
> - Negotiable – based on changing circumstances.
>
> Roles in an organisation can be managed by:
>
> - Negotiating role expectations;
> - Recognising that role security is important but so is role change;
> - Negotiating role change for managers and staff.

Reflection

Many experienced managers will try to ensure that they shape their jobs to 'play' to their own strengths and 'play down' their weaknesses. For example, if they have an expertise in financial matters they will make this their priority and, if possible, their main objective when they are being appraised.

1. Reflect on the behaviour of any experienced managers who you have worked with. Did they make their jobs their own? How did they overcome their weaknesses? (See Negotiating Job Content.)

Managers' roles

There are four main roles that managers undertake in organisations.

Control

The method used by managers to control the work of others in organisations depends on the type of organisation, the role and the job descriptions of people who work for it. For example, factories may expect their workers to clock on, whereas professionals do not expect to have to use a time card. In organisations employing professionals it is not unusual for there to be an expectation that the professionals will work longer than their paid hours to ensure their jobs are completed.

Lead

While managers are expected to lead, they do not have to be leaders in the classic sense. That is, they may use a co-operative team-based approach rather than taking all decisions themselves, but must be aware that they are ultimately responsible for their workforce. It is vital that they enable their staff to work efficiently, either individually or as a group.

Doers

There is an expectation that managers will supervise, problem solve and negotiate for their department or area, both within and without their immediate sphere of influence. In a clinical setting managers are also expected to have the relevant expertise to be a role model for their team.

Communicator

Attending and chairing meetings is considered part of a manager's role. They are expected to seek and receive information and share it with others. They are considered to be the representative of their department or area, and their team members have an expectation that they will represent their interests in the wider arena (Mintzberg, 1983).

Personality and behaviour

Ultimately the performance of any managerial role will be influenced by a manager's personality and how they perceive their relationship with their workforce. Managers' behaviour will also be influenced by the behaviour of those they work with – their team members and colleagues as well as their own managers. Personality may also be influenced by the organisation and its expectations of a manager's behaviour. Organisations tend to have cultures of their own and what may be acceptable in one organisation may not be condoned in another. The organisation itself can also be influenced by the culture of the society in which it operates.

Key Learning Points

The behaviour of a manager at any one time is the result of:

- Their personality;
- The perception and understanding of others;
- The manager's attitude to the behavioural constraints imposed by the role relationship with others – team members, colleagues, their own manager – as well their attitude to the culture of the organisation;
- The degree to which the manager interacts with others, professionally and socially, with respect to the constraints imposed by their role and by the organisational culture.

Reflection

I first came across diverse cultural expectations when in training. We had some student nurses from a neighbouring hospital seconded to our hospital for clinical experience. When we went to meals in our hospital everyone ate together – first, second and third-year students and the staff nurses. In the hospital that the seconded nurses came from, there was a strict hierarchy. Tables were set aside for the various student intakes, and they were expected to sit on their own tables, strictly segregated by seniority. Their expectations of managerial behaviour were coloured by this culture. For example, they were amazed that our matron knew each of our names and that we expected to be acknowledged individually.

1. Do you accept the culture of the organisation you work for or have you ever made a conscious attempt to change it? (See Negotiating Job Content and Changing Staff Roles, as well as Charles Handy's *Understanding Organizations* (1999).)

Summary of Key Learning Points

Role conflict and ambiguity occur when there is uncertainty about:

- How a role holder's work is evaluated;
- Their scope for advancement;
- Their scope for responsibility;
- Others' expectations of their performance.

Roles in an organisation can be:

- Prescriptive – as shown on a job description;
- Evaluated – in an appraisal;
- Descriptive – based on the actual duties performed;
- Negotiable – based on changing circumstances.

Roles in an organisation can be managed by:

- Negotiating role expectations;
- Recognising that role security is important but so is role change;
- Negotiating role change for managers and staff.

The behaviour of a manager at any one time is the result of:

- Their personality;
- The perception and understanding of others;
- The manager's attitude to the behavioural constraints imposed by the role relationship with others – team members, colleagues, their own manager – as well their attitude to the culture of the organisation;
- The degree to which the manager interacts with others, professionally and socially, with respect to the constraints imposed by their role and by the organisational culture.

CASE STUDIES

These two case studies examine different aspects of the clash between roles and expectations. They are based on real situations but information that might identify people or organisations has been changed or removed. Answering the questions after the case studies will help you to clarify your thinking on the main points, especially if you are in the process of role change. It should be possible to address the questions in these case studies from the contents of the chapter.

Case study 1

Mrs Hilary Jones has been the manager of Elm Tree for the past six months. She started with the company some ten years earlier as a health care assistant. By completing NVQ qualifications she gradually gained promotion and became deputy manager of a sister home. She is well known within the home as being a fun-loving lady who was always 'one of the girls'. Many of her friends work within the home including her best friend who started with the company at the same time and now works as a senior care assistant. Everything is going smoothly until her friend is involved in a drug error. This is not the first time this had happened and the regional manager says that a full disciplinary investigation is required. As Mrs Jones is walking through the home she overhears her friend stating that 'she will be fine as Hilary will look after her'. Mrs Jones has to deal with the situation while maintaining the integrity of her role. One aspect of her role profile is to manage and monitor staff performance and she has to balance this against the risk of disrupting the atmosphere within the home.

1. How could Mrs Jones have avoided this misapprehension about her role? (See Managing Role Expectations and Changing Staff Roles.)

Case study 2

Everidge nursing home is expanding from 70 beds to 90 beds. This involves building an extension to the property. It is estimated that building works will take the better part of a year. Brian, the owner/manager, is young, dynamic and liked by his staff. As he would like to be involved as project manager for the new build, Jane, one of the ward managers, has been promoted to home manager and will manage the home in his absence. However, Brian still lives on site.

Jane is a perfectly competent manager but, very early in the project, tensions start to emerge. It is not uncommon for a member of staff to approach Brian direct for a management decision, despite the fact that it has been made clear that Jane is now home manager. Brian may also be approached if Jane makes a decision that a member of staff does not like.

1. What can be done to resolve this situation? Examine the different options. (See Managing Role Expectations, Role Conflict and Changing Staff Roles.)

Activities

What are the roles of the manager?
1. Use the further reading provided (Role of the Manager) and reflect on your own role as a manager and/or your experience of being managed.

Assess your current role
2. Does your job description reflect the role that you perform in your organisation? Do you find that you do things the way others expect you to?
3. Reflect on the difficulties that could arise if you were promoted internally. How can they be overcome? (This may have already happened to you so, if it has, reflect back on the experience.)
4. Reflect on your strengths and weaknesses as a manager (or as an aspiring manager). How could you change your job to suit your strengths and weaknesses?
5. Reflect on your own role. Is it clear in all respects? If not, what is ambiguous and why is it ambiguous?

FURTHER READING

Role of the Manager

Buchanan, D. and Huczynski, A. (2004) *Organizational Behaviour* 5th edn., Prentice Hall

This text provides a good explanation of role conflict and how it occurs.

Handy, C. (1999) *Understanding Organizations*. Penguin

Handy relates roles to the wider context of the organisation and explains roles in the context of the culture of the organisation.

Iles, V. (1997) *Really Managing Health Care*. Open University Press

Iles' work examines the relationship between appraisal and role change.

Martin, V. and Henderson, E. (2001) *Managing in Health and Social Care*. Routledge

This text discusses roles in health and social care in a clear and understandable format.

Stewart, R. (1997) *The Reality of Management*. Pan Books

This text is a clear and practical guide to the real issues of managing roles.

Chapter 2

Managing reflective practice and clinical supervision

INTRODUCTION

This chapter will enable you to address National Occupational Standards F3 'Manage continuous quality improvement' and C10 'Develop teams and individuals'. In this chapter you will:

- consider theories and definitions of reflection and clinical supervision;
- compare models of reflection and modes of clinical supervision;
- consider the use of action planning in implementing changes in practice;
- examine strategies for embedding reflective practice and clinical supervision in your workplace;
- examine the issues involved with contracts and recording reflection.

DEFINITIONS AND THEORIES OF REFLECTION AND CLINICAL SUPERVISION

Reflection

Reflection originated as a learning theory and this is still its main function. A reflective practitioner learns from their practice. One of the first people to specifically identify reflection as a way to learn was Dewey (1933). He viewed reflection as 'an active, persistent and careful consideration of any belief or supposed form of knowledge …' (p. 9). Boud *et al.* (1988) stated that 'Reflection … is a generic term for those intellectual and affective activities in which individuals engage to explore their experiences in order to lead to new understandings …' (p. 19). Palmer *et al.* (1994) suggest that 'reflection is far more than a thoughtful approach … it is more a way of being, a state of mind, it is not a passive contemplation, but an active process' (p. 89). There are many more definitions but some generally agreed principles of reflection are identified in these quotes: reflection is active learning by exploring experience leading to new understandings.

Clinical supervision

The NHS Management Executive defined clinical supervision as:

> ... a formal process of professional support and *learning* which enables individual practitioners to develop knowledge and competence, assume responsibility for their own practice and enhance consumer protection and safety of care in complex situations. It is central to the process of learning and to the scope of the expansion of practice and should be seen as a means of encouraging self-assessment and analytical and reflective skills.
>
> (DoH (1993), p. 3)

Reflective practice and clinical supervision

Clinical supervision and reflective practice can interact together in a virtuous circle that can lead to an overall improvement in the quality of care. A virtuous circle occurs when different elements combine to support and enhance each other. For example, clinical supervision encourages reflective practice and reflective practice and learning from practice enhances clinical supervision (see Figure 1). One must support the other so, without reflection, clinical supervision could reinforce bad practice and, without supervision, reflection could lead to individual learning but that learning may not be disseminated to others. The purpose of clinical supervision is to learn from colleagues.

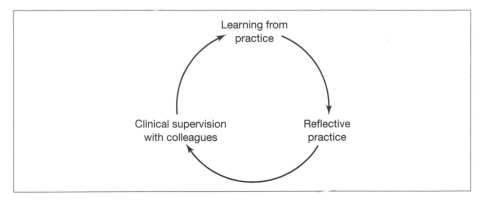

Figure 1 The reflection and clinical supervision virtuous circle

MODELS OF REFLECTION AND MODES OF CLINICAL SUPERVISION

Models of reflection

Most models of reflection are based on a cycle of stages that starts with an observed experience or an event (see Figure 2). We reflect on the event both at the time, that is 'reflection *in* action', and then later, which is 'reflection *on* action' (Kolb, 1984). Thinking about the event takes place immediately (reflection in action) and after the event (reflection on action), and we may reflect and modify our actions as a result.

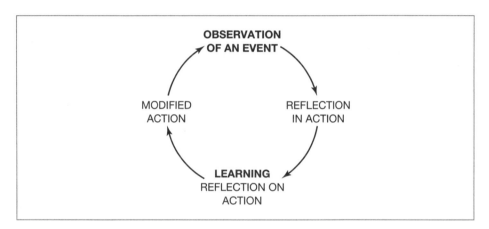

Figure 2 Interpretation of Kolb (1984) – the reflective cycle

The contribution of clinical supervision to reflection is to explore our 'reflections in action' with the supervision group and, with the aid of the supervisor and/or colleagues, to then 'reflect on action'. The immediate learning that occurs when we encounter a situation is shared with the group and may be confirmed or modified.

Johns' model of structured reflection

Johns' model is particularly favoured by health and social care workers as it was developed from practice. Johns envisaged the model being used within a process of guided reflection that includes clinical supervision and the maintenance of a reflective diary (Jasper, 2003). The model has been developed over time but the structure includes two key elements.

A) The core question.
B) Cue questions to promote detailed reflection.

The essence of the model is to uncover and make explicit the knowledge that we use in practice (Johns, 1994, cited in Palmer *et al.*, 1994).

A) The core question

What information do I need to access in order to learn from this experience?

B) Cue questions relating to five key aspects of the experience

1. Description of the experience.
   - What factors contributed to the experience? (Causes)
   - What are the background factors? (Context)
   - What are the key processes in the experience? (Clarifying)
2. Reflection.
   - What was I trying to achieve?
   - What did I do?
   - What were the consequences for myself, the client and their family, colleagues?
   - How did I feel?
   - How did the client feel?
   - How do I know how the client felt?
3. Influencing factors.
   - What internal factors influenced my decision making?
   - What external factors influenced my decision making?
   - What sources of knowledge did/should have influenced my decision making?
4. Could I have dealt with the situation better?
   - What other choices did I have?
   - What would be the consequences of these choices?
5. Learning.
   - How do I feel now about this experience?
   - Can I make sense of it in light of past experiences?
   - What did I learn? (Palmer *et al.*, 1994)

The What Model

Johns' model is used for detailed analysis after the experience is over. The What Model can be used for more immediate analysis:

- **What**   Return to the experience
- **So What**   Understand the experience
- **Now What**   Modify future actions

(Driscoll, 2000)

There is some commonality between Kolb's model, Johns' model and The What Model. All reflective models start from an experience or observation and work towards understanding and learning from experience. The reflection process can be enhanced by colleagues sharing experiences through the process of formal clinical supervision.

Reflection

My main experience of reflective practice is through students' experiences. Their use of a model to examine an experience in depth can be a revelation. A student used Johns' model to examine an unpleasant encounter with a relative. The model enabled her both to understand the experience and to cope with the stress it had caused her. The learning that ensued enabled her to deal with future experiences.

1. Take one recent experience and analyse it using one of the models presented above. What did you learn? (See Models of Reflection.)

Enabling reflective practice

Diaries

Keeping a reflective diary encourages reflective practice. A simple format would be your feelings and thoughts at the time, that is 'reflection in action', and your feelings and thoughts after the incident, that is 'reflection on action'.

Reflective accounts

When you are compiling your practice portfolio a reflective account will illuminate the meaning of the evidence presented. The reflective account can be based on a reflective model such as Kolb's reflective cycle.

Clinical supervision

As is emphasised throughout this chapter, clinical supervision is an excellent strategy for enabling reflective practice.

Critical incidents

Critical incident technique is based on the work of Benner (1984), who states that this is how practitioners develop from novice to expert. Critical incident analysis is one of the many tools that enable reflective practice. A critical incident is:

- an incident in which you felt your intervention/involvement really made a difference either directly or indirectly;
- an incident that went unusually well;
- an incident which did not go as planned;
- an incident that is very ordinary and typical;
- an incident that was particularly demanding.

Critical incident technique reminds us that practitioners can learn from both incidents that go well and from everyday practice. Supervisors should encourage participants to present every kind of incident and not just focus on crises and problems.

Reflection

When I was a 'new' nurse an experienced colleague and I took an elderly client to the bathroom for an assisted bath. I prepared the hoist and started to help the client into it. My colleague said, 'Stop! We don't do anything until we check the temperature of the bath water.' She checked and it was quite cold. I had not realised how long it had been since the bath was filled. The cold water would have been an unpleasant experience for the client. I learned to always check the temperature of the water just before the client went in – a small but important learning experience.

1. Identify the incidents that occur during one day's practice and then classify them according to the criteria above. What did you learn from them? (See Critical Incidents.)

Modes of clinical supervision

Modes of clinical supervision include:

- Individual – meeting one to one with a more experienced clinician acting as supervisor;
- Peer – meeting one to one with an equally experienced clinician;
- Group (led) – meeting as a group with a more experienced clinician acting as supervisor;
- Group (peer) – meeting as a group of people with a similar level of experience, with no designated supervisor or group leader;
- Network – groups of supervisors and supervisees in a contact network (could be phone, e.mail, internet, etc.).

Individual

One-to-one supervision can be an intense experience. It generally involves a newly qualified care professional with a senior care professional acting as supervisor. It is a professional requirement for the professions allied to medicine such as physiotherapy and occupational therapy and is a statutory obligation in child protection work. The Laming Enquiry (2003) that took place after the death of Victoria Climbié (who, despite being known to the social services, died from neglect and abuse) identified the lack of supervision of staff as a major factor. Following the enquiry all child protection workers must now participate in recorded and regular one-to-one clinical supervision. It is very likely that the recommendations for the protection of vulnerable adults, which will apply to all vulnerable adults over eighteen including the elderly, will also include a supervision requirement (Department of Health and the Home Office, 2000).

Individual peer supervision

One-to-one supervision can also include agreed meetings between equally experienced clinicians. Peer supervision can provide support for clinical supervisors.

Group (led) supervision

Group (led) supervision groups are the favoured mode of supervision used in most NHS Trusts. The leader is usually an experienced professional with some training in clinical supervision, and the group can include anyone who has contact with clients, including care assistants. This mode of supervision is often found in the social care sector. In nurse training Personal Tutor Groups (PTG) often use this method as a way of encouraging students to reflect on incidents that have occurred on their placements. The group leader, the tutor, can provide support and comments.

Peer supervision groups

Peer supervision groups, consisting of equally experienced professionals without a leader, are often cited by care professionals as their favoured mode of supervision. In reality they rarely seem to happen, probably due to the time involved in initiating and developing a group. Led groups can develop into peer groups as the members of the group develop in experience and confidence. Peer supervision groups are appropriate for clinical supervisors to support each other. Similar groups are developed in the management training context. It is not uncommon for students who have attended a management course to continue to meet on a regular basis when the course has finished. These groups can be very supportive and a safe place for managers to discuss and reflect on management problems.

Network supervision

Network supervision uses modern technology to keep scattered care professionals in touch. A network can be sustained with phone calls, e.mail and the internet.

Reflection

I co-ordinate clinical supervision workshops. Members often state that they find led group and one-to-one supervision helpful for their professional development but, as supervisors, they most appreciate the support they get from peer supervision. Many participants in the workshop stay in touch and form networks.

1. If you are managing clinical supervisors how do you support them? If you are setting up clinical supervision groups how will you support them? If you are a clinical supervisor what support would you like? (See Modes of Clinical Supervision.)

The requirement for clinical supervision

In the Health Service a requirement to participate in clinical supervision, either one to one or in a group, is being included in job descriptions and will also be monitored at appraisal. The social care sector does not yet have a formal requirement but Commission for Social Care Inspection (CSCI) Inspectors are now including clinical supervision initiatives in their inspection reports.

Key Learning Points

- Both reflection and clinical supervision are about learning from practice.
- Reflection and clinical supervision interact together to improve quality of care.
- All reflective theories identify experience as their starting point and have learning from experience as their purpose.
- Different modes of clinical supervision can be used according to needs and circumstances.

The processes of supervision

All modes

- Prior to the session the practitioner reflects and records relevant aspects of their practice in relation to their role.

- Supervision sessions occur regularly at set times, during work time. A suitable room should be designated for the purpose and it should be made clear that no one should interrupt the session apart from agreed circumstances such as emergencies.

The processes used during the session are adapted according to the number of participants and their needs.

Led group supervision

In a group with one supervisor and a small group of supervisees, the supervisor facilitates the group and monitors the time. An agreed number of people bring a prepared reflection on practice, based on a clinical incident. Figure 3 shows a suggested timetable for a group of eight people.

One-hour session

10 minutes	Review of previous group
10 minutes	Identify any urgent issues
1 person	**Presenting**
5 minutes	Presentation
10 minutes	Discussion with whole group participating
1 person	**Presenting**
5 minutes	Presentation
10 minutes	Discussion with whole group participating
10 minutes	Review of session, plan next session

Figure 3 Led group supervision timetable

Peer group

All members of the group act in a co-operative way, with no one identified as supervisor. One person monitors the time. Some peer groups rotate the supervisor or co-ordinator role if they want more structured sessions.

One to one

The supervisee brings their reflection on practice to discuss with the supervisor. The supervisor is usually an expert and the supervisee is a novice. The structure is very similar to a group supervision but, with only two people involved, the session would probably last 20–30 minutes.

Elements of supervision

It is important that clinical supervision is regarded as a work-time activity and part of normal duties. The main purposes of clinical supervision are:

- professional development;
- improving competence;
- improving the quality of care.

Supervision is not appraisal or a formal teaching process. There is an overlap with mentoring but it is better to keep the two activities separate, although the same person may be doing both. Mentoring is when a skilled individual acts as a role model for a less-experienced or less-qualified person and it takes place throughout the day. Clinical supervision is an activity with boundaries and a very specific purpose. Similarities between the two include the discussion of care related issues and, of course, learning from practice.

Responsibilities in clinical supervision (Driscoll, 2000)

Supervisee
- Identify pertinent stories from your practice.
- Be aware of what you do in practice.
- Accept constructive feedback from your supervisor and colleagues.

Supervisor
- Establish a safe environment.
- Explore and clarify thinking.
- Share information and experiences.

Key Learning Points

- The process is similar for all modes of supervision.
- Clinical supervision is a work activity.
- Both supervisor and supervisee have responsibilities.

Planning for clinical supervision

Introducing clinical supervision into the workplace is a strategic decision and benefits from a careful planning process. Action planning is a process specifically designed to implement change and will be familiar to health and social care professionals as it is the basis of the care planning process and follows a similar sequence of assessment, planning and evaluation. Change will be dealt with in some detail in Chapter 13 but action planning is one approach to change that suits introducing clinical supervision particularly well.

Action planning

Action planning is based on the change theories of Lewin (1951) and Lippett (1973). While they were devised some time ago, they are very much in current use. Lewin's theory is a very simple stage theory and Lippett gives an explanation of what to do at each stage (see Figure 4).

Lewin	Lippett
Unfreezing	Awareness, analysis, assessment Devise change objectives which should be: • observable; • measurable; • timed.
Moving	Choosing a change agent to 'manage' the change Implement step-by-step change strategies
Refreezing	Maintenance of change Terminate helping relationships

Figure 4 Lewin's and Lippett's change theories

Key Learning Points

- Introducing clinical supervision needs a planned approach and continuous attention.
- Clinical supervision must become part of everyday practice to survive.

A sample action plan for clinical supervision

Assessment

The current situation.

> At the last CSCI Inspection the inspectors asked what arrangement we had in place for clinical supervision. We have been doing this on a one-to-one basis, usually when there has been a critical incident. The inspectors stated that they would like to see something more structured next time they inspect the home.

Objectives

Two realistic objectives.

> 1. Ask staff what they want with regard to clinical supervision.
> 2. Identify potential supervisors and explore options for training.

Strategies

Identify strategies for achieving objectives.

> 1. Call a home meeting to discuss clinical supervision.
> 2. Interview staff concerning their knowledge and experience of clinical supervision. Contact the education managers at the local Trust to see what education and training is available.

Evaluation

Evaluate achievement of strategies.

> Objective (1) not yet achieved. Very little knowledge about clinical supervision among staff – several never heard of it – and we could not get all staff at one meeting so a series of meetings is required.
>
> Objective (2) achieved. Several members of staff have the potential to be supervisors but no one has formal training. The local Trust has workshops on clinical supervision and is happy to invite us to participate in these.

Management strategies for embedding clinical supervision in the workplace

Policies

A clinical supervision policy is very important. Wherever possible it should be agreed by all and supported by management. Key elements of the policy include an agreement covering:

- the definition of clinical supervision;
- the number of hours for supervision, e.g. six sessions per year;
- work time should be used, wherever possible;
- the strategy for ensuring all can participate – provision is made for part-time staff and night-duty staff, e.g. remuneration or time back if they come for supervision in their own time;
- the mode of supervision;
- the contract and record-keeping.

Ground rules

Ground rules are very important. They should be set by the group at the initial session as this encourages group involvement. Ground rules generally are of two types, practical and ethical.

- **Practical rules** include things like when meetings take place, for how long, how many presenters there will be and the timetable. They can also include issues such as refreshments, and who to contact if you cannot make a meeting or are going to be late.
- **Ethical rules** include confidentiality and consideration for others. For example, no rudeness, no talking over each other.

The above are just suggestions. Each group should agree on what ground rules are acceptable and relevant to them. Ground rules should be reviewed on a regular basis. If a group is having difficulties, a review of the rules can rectify the situation and help the group understand why the problems are occurring. Regular reviews can also ensure that the group remains focused on learning from practice and improving the quality of care.

Key Learning Points

- There must be agreed policy and management support.
- Ground rules are important.

Sample contracts and clinical supervision records

Contract

Supervisor agrees to:

- establish a safe environment;
- explore and clarify thinking;
- share information and experiences.

Supervisee agrees to:

- identify pertinent stories from my practice;
- be aware of what I do in practice;
- accept constructive feedback from supervisor and colleagues.

(Driscoll, 2000)

Date and Times

We will meet every eight weeks at an agreed time and place. The dates and times of meetings for this year (contract will be reviewed on a yearly basis) are:

1. _____
2. _____
3. _____
4. _____
5. _____
6. _____

Records

Both supervisor and supervisee will keep records in the agreed format. Records will be confidential except in the case of unsafe, unethical or illegal activity. Discussions regarding problematic activities can take place outside the meeting but, wherever possible, this should only be with the supervisee's consent.

Supervisee

I will attend meetings on the agreed dates or send apologies with an explanation of why I cannot attend.

Supervisor

I will arrange meetings and venues as appropriate and will contact the group and/or arrange a substitute supervisor if I cannot lead the group on an agreed date.

Signature of Supervisee _____

Signature of Supervisor _____

Date of Contract _____   Date of Review _____

Supervisor's Record Form   Date _____

Names of Group _____

Attendees _____

_____

_____

Apologies _____

_____

_____

Key Issues Discussed

1. _____

2. _____

3. _____

4. _____

Group Action Plan

Names   Actions

_____   _____

_____   _____

_____   _____

_____   _____

Supervisee's Record Form

Name _____ Date _____

Key Issues

1. _____

2. _____

3. _____

4. _____

Individual Action Plan _____

Personal Reflection _____

Summary of Key Learning Points

- Both reflection and clinical supervision are about learning from practice.
- Reflection and clinical supervision interact together to improve quality of care.
- All reflective theories identify experience as their starting point and have learning from experience as their purpose.
- Different modes of clinical supervision can be used according to needs and circumstances.
- The process is similar for all modes of supervision.
- Clinical supervision is a work activity.
- Both supervisor and supervisee have responsibilities.
- Introducing clinical supervision needs a planned approach and continuous attention.
- Clinical supervision must become part of everyday practice to survive.
- There must be agreed policy and management support.
- Ground rules are important.

Case study

Mr Harris is a qualified nurse who has studied basic psychology as part of his own professional development. In line with recommendations from the Nursing and Midwifery Council, he wants to encourage an environment in which qualified nurses have time to reflect on practice and then use experiential learning. This was discussed with all the trained staff and they agreed to read literature on the Johns' Model of Reflection (1995). It was agreed that this would be tied to six supervision sessions. At the first supervision session the ground rules were decided. Staff would be encouraged to write reflective accounts of critical incidents. These would then be discussed in detail, key issues identified and action plans developed that would include training/development needs. Over the year the staff developed a reflective diary. The manager had been able to link concerns about individual practice issues to the discussions so areas were addressed in an open way which was not destructive. By the end of the year the manager had a much better picture of the individual strengths within the team and could allocate roles appropriately. The staff also had a reflective document that they could put into their portfolios. Staff found this a positive way of using the supervision sessions that they had previously seen as an imposition on their valuable time.

1. How would you set up a clinical supervision group?
2. Would you do it differently if the group was one of care assistants rather than qualified staff?

Activities

1. Are you a reflective practitioner? If you had to present evidence of reflective practice, how would you do this?
2. What do you understand by clinical supervision? How do you undertake it – on your own, in a group, in a formal setting or whenever and wherever it is convenient?
3. You are setting up clinical supervision in your care home. What mode of supervision would you use and why?
4. Assess your care environment. What needs to be changed and why? Identify two initial change objectives.
5. The senior care assistants and managers have been asked to write a clinical supervision policy. What would you include under the following headings?
   - A definition of clinical supervision.
   - Agreed hours for supervision, e.g. six sessions per year.
   - How to ensure it is a work-time activity and how to deal with part-time and night workers.
   - Sample contract and records; see above for examples.

Chapter 3

Decision making

INTRODUCTION

The topic of decision making will enable you to address National Occupational Standard A4: 'Contribute to improvements at work'.

In this chapter you will:

- consider theories and definitions of decision making;
- use a framework for decision making to understand your organisation;
- apply decision-making models to your practice;
- consider different approaches to problem solving;
- consider the use and application of decision-making tools;
- consider staff development regarding decision making.

THEORIES AND DEFINITIONS OF DECISION MAKING

'Decision making is the process of choosing among alternatives and implementing an approach to deal with the problem' (Broody, 2005, p. 84). Broody regards decision making as the partner of problem solving and states that distinctions between the two are artificial. Decision making, in his view, is the action phase of problem solving.

Charles Handy's (1999) view of decision making is that it differs according to the culture of the organisation involved. The following is an interpretation of Handy's work related to decision making. There are four types of organisational culture.

- The power culture.
- The role culture.
- The task culture.
- The person culture.

The power culture

The power culture is frequently found in small entrepreneurial organisations. Decision making is accelerated as the only person to convince is the leader of the organisation. The leader has the authority to change the organisation. This can be effective and efficient but if the decision is a poor one there is no way to discuss decisions and their outcomes.

The role culture

The role culture is dependent on rules and procedures. The job description delineates the individual's authority or lack of authority to make decisions. As long as the decision is straightforward and relates to the individual's role, problems are minimised and the decision taker is protected by the system. If a decision is risky and not covered by the role, the system may withdraw its protection. This type of system does not encourage any risk taking, which can be a disadvantage in times of rapid change.

The task culture

In the task culture decisions are based on the expertise of the decision maker. The task culture focuses on the job or product, and the basis of the organisation is the team or the group. Decisions are made co-operatively.

The person culture

The true person culture is rare; legal chambers and GP practices are two examples of person cultures. Decisions are made by autonomous individuals who are wholly responsible for the decision and the results of the decision.

Nursing and residential care homes plus long-stay units in the health service can take on characteristics of any of these cultures. A privately owned nursing home may be a power culture or a role culture depending on the preferences or personality of the owner, whereas a specialist team in a hospital-based long-stay unit may take on the characteristics of a task culture. See below in 'A Framework for Decision Making' for clues to the culture you work in.

A FRAMEWORK FOR DECISION MAKING

Decision making is considered part of a manager's job. You should know from your systems at work:

- what you can or cannot decide;
- when a decision should be made;
- the information necessary to make decisions;
- ways to get decisions implemented.

Handy (1999, p. 215) states that decisions in an organisation can be made by the person:

- with the higher power or authority (Power Culture);
- whose job description carries the responsibility (Role Culture);
- who has the most knowledge and expertise about the problem (Task Culture);
- most involved and affected by the outcome (Person Culture).

What kind of culture do you work in? Who makes the decisions?

Managers have four decisional roles:

1. Entrepreneur – they make the business decisions for their area/department;
2. Disturbance handler – manage conflicts that arise;
3. Resource allocator – resources that include the manager's time (often forgotten);
4. Negotiator – with staff, other managers and outside agencies as well as patients/clients.

Time span

The managerial level at which decisions are made in an organisation has a relationship to the time in which the outcome is likely to be seen. At the top level (chief executive, Trust board, nursing home owner), management makes strategic decisions. Strategic plans are usually for three to five years ahead but, as all spheres of life are changing at a rapid rate, most strategic plans are updated annually. (Strategic decision making will be considered in Chapter 15.)

Middle management makes decisions that will influence the next two to three months, while first-line management makes the day-to-day decisions. This is not to say that first-line managers do not make strategic decisions. They do, but their job is to keep the organisation running on a daily basis. The results of decision making at lower levels can be more readily seen as they take place over a shorter period of time, fewer factors may need to be taken into account, and the stages of decision making can be telescoped in time.

Reflection

The time line of decision making is taken into account by the trade unions when they go out on strike. Few managers ever go on strike because, if they do, they are unlikely to be missed for a while. However, front-line workers are missed from the time they go on strike.

1. What is your level in your organisation? If you were to be absent from your organisation how long would it be before a decision had to be made that only you could make? (See above on A Framework for Decision Making and Theories and Definitions of Decision Making.)

The decision-making link with time spans can have other consequences if the results of your decision will not be evident for a while. You can retire or move to another job, and it is then difficult to be held accountable for any subsequent problems. Time can also deter decision making. If you leave things long enough you may not have to make a decision as you may have moved or the problem will have been resolved. These factors may have influenced strategic planning in the health and social services over time.

Reflection

During the NHS reorganisation in the 1990s contracting for nurse education was introduced at the same time that radical managerial changes occurred. The numbers of nurses who were recruited into training declined. By the turn of the century it was evident that the country had insufficient nurses and large numbers of overseas nurses were recruited. The managers who had made the original decisions to decrease the numbers in training had long since retired or moved to other jobs. Something similar appears to be happening now based on economic factors and this will also have implications for the future.

1. When you make a decision, within what time span can you be held accountable for the consequences? (See above on Time spans.)

Key Learning Points

Decision making is influenced by:

- The culture of the organisation;
- The role of the manager;
- The time span related to the type of decision.

USING AND APPLYING MODELS OF DECISION MAKING

Steps in decision making

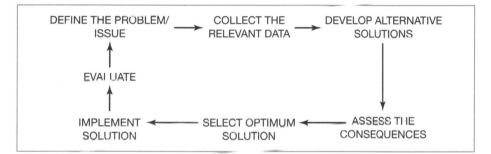

Figure 1 A decision model (adapted from Cole, 1990, p. 109)

Define the problem

It is important when making a decision that the problem is defined accurately. It is quite a common mistake for managers to think they know what the problem is, but the cause of the problem may have changed, problems can be too narrowly defined or the cause was never what it was assumed to be and information can be wrong. Also, all managers should know the problems that their staff are dealing with, but there is an inclination to ignore problems. What tends to happen is that:

- if a problem is not obvious it is not a problem;
- if a problem has not happened before it is not going to happen.

Reflection

Within many care homes there is a consistent problem with providing individualised continence care. Most people accept that it is in all residents' interests to have their own continence products. One way of achieving this is to keep each resident's products within their rooms. This regularly leads to staff using them for other clients because they are more easily available. As a result, homes regularly run out of products before the next delivery is due. The staff will then complain that there are no wipes, pads or gloves.

1. Reflect on the possible reasons why commonplace and apparently simple problems appear never to be solved. Do you have any similar problems in your organisation? (See A Framework for Decision Making and Charles Handy's work on organisational cultures (Handy, 1999)).

Problems can be more complex than anticipated and analysis may take more time than anticipated.

Reflection

All health and social care environments involved in the transfer of care of older people face dilemmas around the safe but timely discharge of patients/residents. They are also faced with what can sometimes be seen as contradictory targets set by government bodies. Care home and hospital staff may well be in agreement about the need to reduce hospital admissions but this can often mean different things to individuals. A discharge facilitator may define this in terms of ensuring that clients are assessed and, if they need residential care, that they are placed as quickly as possible. A care home representative may feel that time should be taken to allow the patient to be actively involved in making the decision, even if this means taking longer. It is felt that if the client is actively involved they are less likely to be readmitted due to a failed discharge.

1. If you were a decision maker in either type of organisation, what would be your priorities in solving these opposite but related problems? (See Cole's decision model above and Defining the problem.)

Collect the information

It is not uncommon for decisions to be made despite a lack of sufficient information needed to make them. In an emergency this can be acceptable. Sometimes a decision has to be made which is not the best one. In non-emergency situations there is no excuse for not setting aside the time to collect the information needed to analyse the problem. Also, care must be taken to collect accurate information, as a solution based on inaccurate data may cause more difficulties later.

Reflection

I was once asked to complete an employee's questionnaire that asked how I got to work. In those days I cycled. When I returned the completed questionnaire to the secretary she read my replies and commented that I shouldn't have filled in the questionnaire as I didn't have a car. The questionnaire was about how staff got to work because the firm wanted to know what people did so they could make provision for them e.g. car parking spaces. The secretary had decided that it was only for car drivers and so had handed it out only to them which meant that bicycle parking spaces were unlikely to be provided.

1. What went wrong in the chain of command to allow the above to happen? (See A Framework for Decision Making.)

Identify the options

It is important to ensure that you do not only look at the obvious solutions; there may be other options, as for example with the car users Reflection above. If the decision has a direct effect on other staff, then encouraging them to suggest possible solutions could be helpful.

Assess the consequences

The consequences of each possible solution must be tested or weighed. It may be that all possible solutions to a problem have consequences in, for example, a 'no win' situation, in which case a decision to limit any 'damages' may be the most sensible option. It may be that the choice between the different options is no choice, but that there is a path of least resistance, with limited damage.

Determine the best alternative

Having tested and weighed the consequences, you need to decide on the best solution. It must be remembered that a decision made in one set of circumstances may not be ideal in another. It can sometimes help to use numbers and data to make a decision and a quantitative ranking table (see Figure 2) can be used.

Alternatives	Cost	Risk	Time	Resources
A				
B				
C				

Figure 2 A quantitative ranking table

Reflection

We had over 50 suitable candidates for a ten-place Enrolled Nurse conversion course. To decide on the first 10 students we allocated points for age (there was a cut-off age), date of application, time with employer, academic work, etc. The students were ranked and the top 10 came on the first course. As the courses were ongoing, we could also give the students who were unsuccessful the first time around an idea of when they would be put on a course, and they were also made aware of the criteria used for the decisions.

1. Try using a table when you next have to make a decision at work or at home. You will need to decide on your own criteria and give them values. The following is an example of using a ranking table to assess the risk of fire in a care home (see Figure 3).

Risk of fire in a care home

Alternatives	Cost	Risk	Time	Resources
A. Do no fire training	None	**High**. If a fire does occur, there could be loss of life, injuries and extensive damage.	None	None

B. Do initial fire training on induction	6 hours staff pay 6 hours pay for tutor	Staff will have some knowledge, which may become dated after time. Less likely to take pre-emptive action as part of everyday work. If a fire does occur, could still have loss of life.	4 hours	Tutor Equipment Room
C. Carry out initial fire training and annual up-dates	6 hours pay for all staff 6 hours pay for tutor for each 10 staff members	All staff will be aware of risk of fire and should take pre-emptive action whenever necessary. If a fire does occur, loss of life and injuries should be preventable and at worst minimal.	6 hours each member of staff	Tutor Equipment Room

Figure 3 A quantitative ranking table assessing the risk of fire in a care home

Reflection A

Drivers often have to make split-second decisions. If a car is heading directly for you in a limited space, do you hit it straight on? Try to deflect to one side? Or head to the hard shoulder if there is one? None of these alternatives will prevent damage, but you could sustain less damage.

Reflection B

As the manager of a home you are asked to take a resident on a short-term placement. The resident is currently living at home alone and is above the normal level of dependence for your home. The care manager has indicated that there are no local alternative placements and the resident has refused hospitalisation. After assessing the risk to the resident and your home, do you admit the prospective resident?

1. Use the quantitative ranking table above to work out the best solution for the above scenarios.

Decision tree

Another tool to help decide between different solution options is a decision tree (see Figures 4 and 5). This is often called an algorithm, the principle of which is sometimes used when making a medical diagnosis. Decision trees can be useful in helping to focus decision making. An example can be found at **www.mindtools.com/dectree.html**.

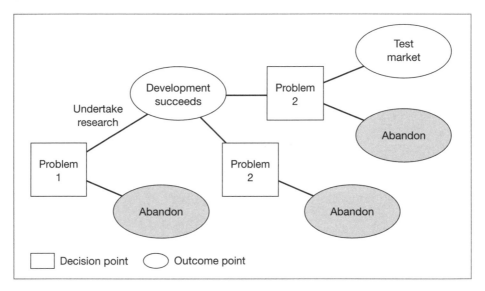

Figure 4 A decision tree (adapted from Cole, 1990, p. 168)

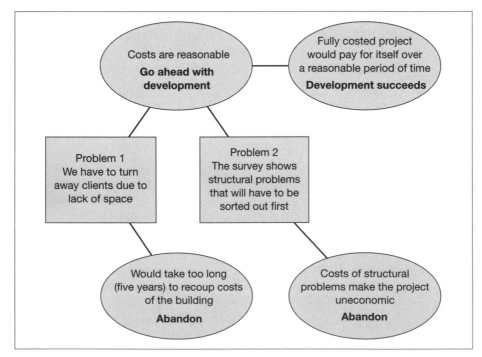

Figure 5 A decision tree for extending a care home

Act and evaluate

Having acted on a decision, you should then evaluate the outcomes. It is a common mistake to make a decision and not evaluate the outcomes, only to find that later the same problem or another related to the decision is still occurring. It must be remembered that it takes time to make good decisions and to evaluate the consequences.

Other factors to consider when making decisions

It is important to take the following factors into consideration when making decisions.

Rationality

Is one solution more likely to be rational than another? It is important to examine the likely consequences of a decision when considering its rationality. A decision that appears rational may have unintended consequences.

Reflection

A Trust wanted to bring some elective orthopaedic patients onto the main site. To accommodate these patients other patients needed to be moved to what had been the orthopaedic hospital two miles away. It was decided that it would be appropriate to move a ward of elderly care patients. Those making the decision did not appreciate that all the patients in the elderly care ward were admitted for treatment of acute conditions. They assumed they did not need the investigative facilities of a main hospital. It was not until the x-ray manager pointed out that every patient admitted invariably had at least one x-ray, which would require an ambulance transfer to the main site after the move, that it was decided to transfer day surgery beds instead.

1. Did the managers have enough information to make a rational decision?
2. Apply the decision tree to this scenario. Would it have helped the managers to make their decision?

Trustworthy information

It is sometimes difficult to assess the trustworthiness of information. This is particularly the case when the parties involved in the decision have vested interests or are using inaccurate or even fraudulent information.

Acceptance of the decision made

Is the acceptance of the decision by subordinates important for implementation? While some subordinates will always go along with the manager's decisions regardless, it is a sensible manager who takes subordinates' views into account. Decision making can be improved when decisions have to be justified.

Evaluating decisions and retaining control

There can be an inherent dislike of analysing decisions. Often wishes, hopes and internal politics play a part in a final decision. Decision making is usually made in a hurry with inadequate information and, even after analysis and evaluation, there may be no agreement as to the consequences of the decision. If there is a disagreement, there is likely to be a compromise or alternatively no action taken at all. Remember that if subordinates do not agree with a decision they may well either consciously or unconsciously sabotage the outcomes. Managers need to retain control over the decision-making process. Mintzberg (1983) shows that the decision-making process can be influenced at a number of stages (see Figure 6).

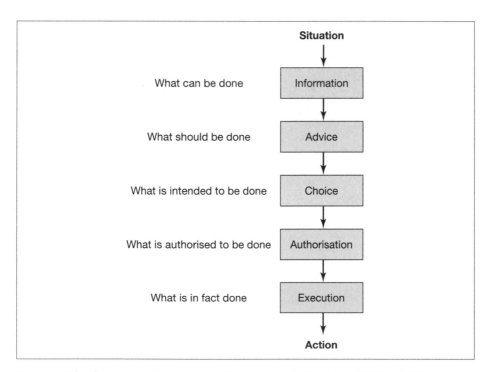

Figure 6 The decision-making action-taking process (Mintzberg, 1983, p. 114)

> **Key Learning Points**
>
> Models of decision making can help to:
>
> - Define the problem;
> - Develop alternative solutions;
> - Select the best solution;
> - Evaluate the consequences.

STAFF DEVELOPMENT

The differences in the types of decision making at different levels in an organisation have implications for recruitment, training and promotion. It is difficult to give managers training in decision making as the type of training will depend on the type, frequency and rapidity with which decisions have to be made in the job. Some personalities thrive on making quick decisions as, for example, they need to in the emergency services. Others find it difficult and stressful to make decisions even over a period of time. Training can be given and managers can delegate decision making in order to provide learning situations.

The quality of decision making can be improved by understanding the environment in which the organisation works. Decision making can also vary depending on the type of organisation. For example, decision making will be different in profit-making businesses, public services and charities. In public services politics may play a larger role than it does in a profit-making organisation. Public service organisations may also be more restricted by legislation and ethical considerations than a profit-making business.

It is essential that members of staff are taught to analyse the available information at each step of the process as well as evaluate decisions that they have made. However, while care staff can be taught to use decision models, assess uncertainties and examine the effects of making different assumptions in theory, their behaviour may actually be very different in a real situation where the consequences may be life threatening. To facilitate their decision-making abilities, staff need to be given the opportunity to develop the confidence to make decisions. It can be helpful to give junior staff opportunities to take charge even though their manager is present and on duty. This demonstrates that you have confidence in their ability to cope and make decisions. If they make a decision that the manager does not agree with, then the staff member should evaluate the decision they made with the manager. The manager is still ultimately accountable for any decisions made in this learning situation, so they need to understand how the junior staff member came to his or her decision. After all, it may be that the staff member has taken factors into account that the manager was not aware of, or had not thought of, and the decision they made is in fact better than that the manager would have made. Alternatively, the manager may have to explain exactly why the decision was unsuitable. As this is a learning situation, it is important to ensure the staff member does not lose confidence during the exercise.

Reflection

As a manager there is a temptation to make all the decisions yourself. It is quicker and, of course, you have the experience to make better decisions. However, it is an important part of staff development that they should learn to make decisions themselves, otherwise the situation of the 'manager in the morning' is liable to develop, i.e. when the manager is off duty, junior staff will not make decisions but will leave them for the 'manager in the morning'. I am sure you will recognise situations where, when you come back on duty, there are a lot of problems to sort out that could have been dealt with by the staff on duty at the time.

1. Using the information in this section on staff development, how can you ensure that your junior staff are willing and able to make decisions?

Key Learning Points

Decision-making abilities can be developed at all levels by:

• Training and delegation;
• Encouraging the analysis of information;
• Encouraging the evaluation of decisions;
• Confidence building.

Summary of Key Learning Points

Decision making is influenced by:

• The culture of the organisation;
• The role of the manager;
• The time span related to the type of decision.

Models of decision making can help to:

- Define the problem;
- Develop alternative solutions;
- Select the best solution;
- Evaluate the consequences.

Decision-making abilities can be developed at all levels by:

- Training and delegation;
- Encouraging the analysis of information;
- Encouraging the evaluation of decisions;
- Confidence building.

Case study 1

Ambleside is an 80-bed care home with nursing and has been open for ten years. Mr Clark has been the registered manager for the past five years. In a recent CSCI inspection the home received a recommendation related to Standard 27 of the National Minimum Care Standards. The inspectors felt that, due to the nature of dependency, the current staffing levels on one of the units were no longer adequate. Mr Clarke is aware that his budget currently will not allow for more staff so he needs to consider the options available to him. Some of these options are listed below.

- He has a meeting with his staff to discuss the issue and asks them to feedback with ideas about how they might act differently so that they can use their time more effectively.
- He develops a business plan, in line with his company's overall strategy, which looks at possible savings within the home that may allow release of funds for extra staffing.
- He discusses with staff representatives and union representatives the possibility of changing shift times to enable more staff to be available at busier times of the day.
- He asks his senior staff nurse to read the literature. Other organisations may have found solutions which may be feasible in this situation.

All of these options will be difficult for him as the manager and are also likely to take time. As discussed in this chapter, all alternative solutions may have consequences.

1. Identify the possible consequences, both positive and negative, for each of these solution options.
2. Considering the decision-making framework, which of the four cultures does each solution option fall into?

Case study 2

Mrs Jackson is an assistant manager at a care home owned by a small company that owns four homes. These homes have a good reputation and have received good inspection reports for a number of years. All four homes use a set care plan and Mrs Jackson's home has received fours* for this care plan in the last two inspections. However, the company has recently been taken over by a larger organisation with over 30 care homes and various other facilities. This organisation has always insisted on all their homes using the same paperwork. However, none of the larger organisation's homes have ever received a four for their care plans. All Mrs Jackson's staff are unhappy with the new care plans and feel they are not of the quality of the ones they currently use. The new company is in the process of reviewing its paperwork and has asked for a representative from each geographic area to carry out this work. Mrs Jackson has been chosen as she developed the previous care plan and is quite assertive. Mrs Jackson's manager has stated that this is the best opportunity they have for getting their care plans adopted as the new company plans.

1. This is the first opportunity that Mrs Jackson and the staff from the smaller company have had for changing the ethos of the new larger organisation. How should Mrs Jackson approach this task?
2. How can the decision-making tools above help her plan for the meetings?

*CSCI scores 1 to 4 on seven outcomes related to service quality 1 Poor 2 Adequate 3 Good 4 Excellent.

Activities

1. Reflect on what kind of decisions you make at work. Using Handy's list on page 31, analyse why you are making them. (See Theories and Definitions of Decision Making and A Framework for Decision Making.)
2. Think of examples of decisions that you make in each of the manager's roles outlined on page 33. (See A Framework for Decision Making.)
3. Reflect on your own organisation. At what level are strategic decisions made? Does the time it takes to implement these decisions have any influence on the level at which decisions are taken? (See Time span.)
4. How are decisions made in your organisation? Does the process work? If not, why not? If it does work, why does it work? (See Theories and Definitions of Decision Making and A Framework for Decision Making.)
5. Using Figure 6 'Control over the decision-making process' on page 42, reflect on some of the decisions that you have made recently at work and identify the factors that influenced these decisions at each stage in the process. Were you in control of the decision-making process?

FURTHER READING

This management library may prove useful for further information on
problem solving: **www.mapnp.org/library/prsn_prd/decision.htm**

Chapter 4

Leadership

INTRODUCTION

The topic of leadership will enable you to address National Occupational Standard C13 'Manage the performance of teams and individuals'.

In this chapter you will consider:

- definitions and theories of leadership;
- characteristics of leadership;
- problems of leadership;
- the development and support of leaders.

In 1974 a number of British industrialists signed the following advertisement:

> So far as we are concerned three years as an Army Officer can equal three years at University.
>
> Of course, we don't expect a young man fresh from the Army to be fluent in Medieval French Literature or a Master of Microbiology.
>
> But in our experiences as employers, we've found that a Short Service Commission in the Army equips a man to make the change to business management very easily.
>
> For both jobs are concerned with the handling of people and getting the best out of them, often in trying situations.
>
> (Anyone who's had to keep twenty soldiers calm when a crowd is hurling bricks at them will readily agree.)
>
> And to be frank, there's another aspect we like. All managers have to learn the hard way, and this will have been at the Army's expense, not ours.
>
> (*The Times*, 16 June 1974)

DEFINITIONS AND THEORIES OF LEADERSHIP

> Leadership is a social process in which one individual influences the behaviour of others without the use or threat of violence. (Huczynski and Buchanan, 1991, p. 494)

Leaders are needed most in changing times to show others the way, encourage people to follow, and to have a sense of purpose. Leaders are not always managers, though it is easier to lead if you are a manager. Often leadership and management are used interchangeably, but all managers are not leaders nor are all leaders managers. As Stewart (1996, p. 4) says:

> Managers have staff. Leaders have followers: people who recognise and find attractive the leader's sense of purpose. Leaders are those who can get the people with whom they work to be convinced to be co-operators. Leaders make others feel that what they are doing matters and hence make them feel good about their work. You can give a lead from any position, though the more authority you have the more important it is that you should be a good leader.

- **Administrators** carry out policies and maintain stability. They tend to be found in bureaucratic organisations. They are publicly accountable for what they do and they confirm in writing.
- **Managers** direct staff and manage change or improvements. Good managers are not necessarily good administrators.
- **Leaders** point the way and can bring about radical change. They identify and symbolise what is important. To be successful, leaders have to have followers.

Leadership has been studied for well over a century and various theories have been advanced. Each theory has some elements of the truth.

Trait theories

The earliest studies of leadership focused on the personal qualities of leaders or their traits. It was felt that some members of society had innate leadership qualities. While charisma can play a part in leadership, few possess it. Of the lists produced for 'trait theories', there were many differences but a few common features:

- intelligence;
- initiative;
- self-assurance.

Also, in recent studies, 'The helicopter factor', which is the ability to rise above a situation, is another feature of trait theories (Handy, 1999).

Style theories

Many of the leadership studies since the 1950s have centred on the behaviour or style of the leader, and the way in which leadership is exercised. However, Lewin, Lippitt and White (1937) were the original proponents of style theory. It is based on the spectrums of autocratic-democratic and people-centred – task-orientated behaviours. There is evidence that a supportive style of management will improve the motivation and sense of involvement with the organisation by the workforce but that style alone is not enough to create an effective and efficient organisation. Further research in efficiency led to the development of the contingency theories (see below, p. 52).

McGregor and leadership

In 1960 Douglas McGregor concluded that there were two basic assumptions made by managers which underlaid their attitudes and behaviours. He called these assumptions Theory X and Theory Y. These theories were not the result of research, but have been used in research subsequently. There has been an assumption that managers were motivated by one theory when, in reality, aspects of both may be valid.

Theory X assumes:

- the average human dislikes work and will avoid it if possible;
- people must be coerced, controlled, directed or threatened with punishment in order to ensure adequate effort;
- the average human prefers direction, avoids responsibility where possible, has little ambition and is primarily motivated by a desire for security.

Theory Y assumes:

- mental and physical work is as natural as play or rest;
- the average person can exercise self-direction and self-control;
- intrinsic rewards can be obtained by individual effort;
- people will accept and actively seek responsibility under suitable conditions;
- people can use their imagination, ingenuity and creativity to solve organisational problems.

Rensis Likert

Rensis Likert proposed a four-system variation on the task-centred versus people-centred dichotomy.

1. Exploitive-Authoritative

Power and direction are top down, threats and punishments are used, communication and teamwork is poor, with resultant poor productivity.

2. Benevolent-Authoritative

Has some of the characteristics of the previous system but does allow consultation and delegation. Labour turnover and absenteeism is high, though productivity is fair to good.

3. Consultative

Goals are discussed and communication is both ways, from the bottom and from the top. Teamwork is encouraged and rewards are given. Productivity is excellent.

4. Participative

Communication is good; all participate and are committed to the organisational objectives. Productivity is excellent.

Both Likert (1961) and McGregor (1960) were intrinsic theorists. That is, they believed humans gain satisfaction from their work and, if they are given the opportunity to be involved in decision making and have some control over their work life, they will be motivated to be more productive and effective. This theory was developed in opposition to extrinsic theories which state that the primary motivations are salary and promotion and other 'benefits'.

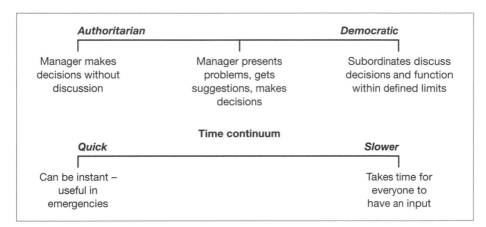

Figure 1 Continuum of leadership styles

While Tannenbaum and Schmidt (1958) proposed a continuum of leadership styles (see Figure 1), they also showed that managers could be flexible and could choose a leadership style. They recognised that not only the manager but the situation and the employees could influence the style that a manager might use. A simplified version of this continuum is still used in managerial interviews and training. Applicants are asked to state where they think they perform best on an Autocratic-Democratic continuum.

Reflection

There is a tendency to feel that democratic leadership is the ideal. However, this may not work in practice. The manager of an Intensive Care Unit retired and the remaining five clinical sisters decided that they would divide the responsibilities between them, with no one being the leader. It lasted about three months. Anyone liaising with the unit found it difficult to get a decision to a managerial problem. The person responsible was often not on duty (the sisters covered all 24 hours in shifts) and no one else would make a decision. After three months one sister was nominated as 'in charge' and the unit ran more smoothly.

1. Care homes often have 'joint leadership', particularly at the assistant manager level. How can this be made to work to avoid the problems identified above? (See Definitions and Theories of Leadership.)

Key Learning Points

Leaders need to be aware of:

- Theories of leadership;
- Their role as a leader;
- Their leadership style.

LEADERSHIP BEHAVIOUR

Contingency theories

Contingency theorists suggested that leadership behaviour was dependent on a wider range of variables. Fiedler (1967) concluded that group performance was dependent on (contingent upon) three main variables:

1. Leader/member relations.
2. The structure of the task.
3. The power and authority of the leader's position.

This could mean that if the leader had little power, was disliked or the task was relatively unstructured, leadership was likely to be ineffective. Other contingency theorists have also suggested that the environment plays a part (see Figure 2).

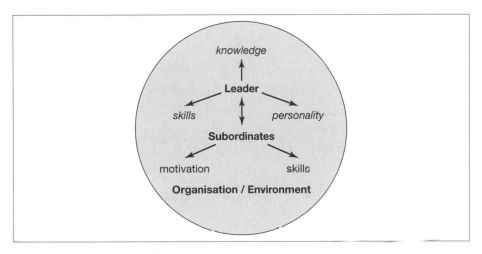

Figure 2 Leadership variables

Adair's (1973) classic functional leadership model (see Figure 3) also has a contingency perspective. There must be a balance between the task and the group and individual needs. This balance will vary and priorities must be decided in each situation. An effective leader is one who sets the priorities correctly. Skills development for leaders is essential.

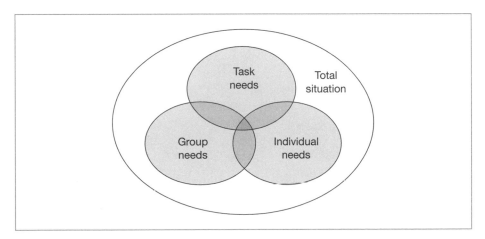

Figure 3 The functional leadership model (adapted from Cole, 1988, p. 50)

Reflection

The balance between the task, the group and the individual needs can mean that leaders will not always be successful in different circumstances. Think of politicians like, for example, Churchill, who was a very popular Prime Minister during the Second World War, but who was voted out of power at the end of the war, when the population felt that they would be better served by a Labour government.

1. Would you be prepared to surrender or share leadership if your particular combination of skills was not suited to a particular task? (See Contingency theories.)

The 'best fit' approach

Handy (1999) developed the idea that the environment was a factor in leadership, as an extension of contingency theory, and suggested six key aspects are involved:

1. The power of the leader.
2. The relationship between the leader and the group.
3. Organisational culture or norms.
4. Structure and technology of the organisation.
5. The variety of tasks.
6. The variety of subordinates.

Handy placed an emphasis on flexibility; the ability to respond to changing circumstances was the hallmark of a good leader. Handy regarded the 'best fit' approach as an extension of contingency theory, with the emphasis on flexibility and the contention that the ability to change in relation to changing circumstances, was the mark of a good leader.

Reflection

On a scale of 1 (low) to 10 (high), what scores would you give to yourself and to your leaders for concern for the task and concern for people?

	Concern for task	Concern for people
Yourself	_____	_____
Your boss	_____	_____

Your boss's boss?   _____   _____

What scores do you
think your colleagues
would give you?   _____   _____

What scores do you
think your boss would
give him/herself?   _____   _____

(Adapted from Martin and Henderson, 2001, p. 53)

CHARACTERISTICS OF LEADERSHIP

Drawing on the theories above, it is possible to identify the characteristics of the good leader.

- Point the way – this can only be done if leaders know what is expected and if they have a vision of what has to be done.
- Symbolise the meaning and the values of the organisation – leaders must show what they care about.
- Leaders can get others to share ideals. In this respect what you do matters more than what you say.
- Leaders create pride in an organisation – the achievement of high standards and enthusiasm for the organisation.
- Leaders make people feel important and thus realise their potential. They need to provide the environment in which people can flourish and develop.
- Leaders must be self-sufficient and self-reliant, as leadership can be lonely and not out to be popular, as they may have to make uncomfortable decisions.
- Leaders need to have a sense of humour.

Key Learning Points

Leaders should consider:

- The needs of the organisation;
- The task to be performed;
- Their legitimate power and authority.

THE PROBLEMS OF LEADERSHIP

Leadership carries inherent problems. Awareness of the pitfalls can help but constant vigilance is needed on the part of the leader. These problems include:

- excessive expectations;
- undue importance attached to your remarks;
- isolation;
- a belief in your own importance;
- lack of confidence.

Reflection

It is easy for undue importance to be attached to a leader's remarks, as Henry II discovered when in a temper he asked 'Who will rid me of this turbulent priest?' and four knights subsequently murdered Archbishop Thomas Becket. Henry of course protested that he did not mean them to murder Thomas. When in a leadership position, care must be taken that comments are not misconstrued.

1. Is it possible to minimise the possibility of such situations arising? What kind of leader do you think Henry II was? (See Characteristics of Leadership and Problems of Leadership.)

THE DEVELOPMENT AND SUPPORT OF LEADERS

Over the last decade there has been an ongoing move to highlight the importance of leadership in all aspects of health and social care. With the development of the Modernisation Agency the Department of Health has provided both actual and virtual support for leaders in a number of clinical areas. The recently updated leadership guides are available to all health and social care environments at **www.wise.nhs.uk**. Although these guides may have been initially written with the National Health Service in mind, the information transfers to other care environments including care homes.

Care homes have been actively involved in leadership projects and one which has been successfully evaluated is the Royal College of Nursing leadership programme for older people's nurses. This programme promotes leadership skills and approaches across the varied settings where older people may be cared for. The programme encourages staff such as matrons, consultant nurses and unit/ward managers to meet together and learn with and from each other. One real strength of the programme is that it encourages a 'buddy' approach for hospital, community and care home staff. Information about the course can be found at **www.rcn.org.uk/development/practice/leadership**. The programme initially announced in April 2005 has seen its first graduates and valuable links have been made between both public and voluntary sector employees. These approaches, along with other programmes such as the Leading in Empowered Organisations programme, are often aimed at people in higher positions within organisations. It is important to consider the point discussed within this section that leaders are not necessarily managers.

Other programmes which have been successful encourage organisations to look more widely for their leaders. Many leaders may already be in staff groups and just need the opportunity to express ideas and lead on specific projects. One such project is the Continuing Professional Development project from Leeds University **www.cdhpp.leeds.ac.uk/services/practice2.php**. This ongoing project encourages units of all types to sign up to become Practice Development Units. Teams are again not restricted by their area of practice and care homes have been actively involved. Through reaching accreditation as a practice development unit, care homes have been encouraged to look to all involved in the life of residents for ideas about how to improve the quality of the units. The aim is that ideas are openly discussed and looked at with a framework tool which enables staff to consider where they are and where they want to be. Within this structure no one person's views are more or less important than those of anybody else.

Within the best units ideas come from residents, relatives and all levels of staff. This enables managers to take a supportive role without having to take over, as well as giving other staff of all grades the chance to lead on projects and come up with workable and affordable solutions. Another advantage is that it also encourages units to look at themselves as being part of local communities and to look at ways they can support institutions such as local schools but also to consider what benefits such relationships may have for the unit. The programme enables the units to develop a relationship with Leeds University through an ongoing teaching and support package and allows the units to promote some of the good work that goes on within care homes. Other universities and institutions have developed similar programmes and this has again been a way for care homes to challenge some of the negative stereotypes that have been associated with them.

> **Key Learning Points**
>
> Leaders should be aware of:
>
> - The inherent problems of leadership;
> - Their need for development;
> - Existing support structures.

CONCLUSION: A LEADER'S PRAYER

Dear Lord, help me to become the kind of leader my management would like to have me be. Give me the mysterious something which will enable me at all times satisfactorily to explain policies, rules, regulations and procedures to my workers even when they have never been explained to me.

Help me teach and to train the uninterested and dim-witted without ever losing my patience or my temper.

Give me that love for my fellow men which passes all understanding so that I may lead the recalcitrant, obstinate, no-good worker into the path of righteousness by my own example, and by soft persuading remonstrance, instead of busting him on the nose.

Instil into my inner-being tranquillity and peace of mind that no longer will I wake from my restless sleep in the middle of the night crying out, 'What has the boss got that I haven't got and how did he get it?'

Teach me to smile if it kills me.

Make me a better leader of men by helping develop larger and greater qualities of understanding, tolerance, sympathy, wisdom, perspective, equanimity, mind-reading and second sight.

And when, Dear Lord, Thou has helped me to achieve the pinnacle my management has prescribed for me and when I shall have become the paragon of all supervisory virtues in this earthly world, Dear Lord, move over, Amen.

(Handy, 1999, p. 98)

Summary of Key Learning Points

Leaders need to be aware of:

- Theories of leadership;
- Their role as a leader;
- Their leadership style.

Leaders should consider:

- The needs of the organisation;
- The task to be performed;
- Their legitimate power and authority.

Leaders should be aware of:

- The inherent problems of leadership;
- Their need for development;
- Existing support structures.

Case study 1

A common problem in many care settings is producing quality person-centred care plans. When they have been developed it is often even more difficult to ensure that they are used. This is an area where traditional management approaches have not always been effective. The example below indicates how a leadership approach helped to transform the care planning within an NHS Continuing Care unit.

Hyburn House is an 18-bed unit within a community hospital which houses clients with very high level care needs. Many of the clients have complex physical and psychological needs. Care planning is often difficult as clients are unable to communicate their needs clearly and sensitive end-of-life decisions have to be made. Managers linked to the unit had tried to influence this by looking at different tools and using clinical audit. Staff had not responded to this so a different approach was tried. The unit manager Mr Grey decided that an approach of group care planning should be tried. This meant gathering small teams within the unit together to discuss an individual's care needs. The teams included nurses and care assistants and the teams were asked to allocate the writing of the care plan to different members. Within the meetings

Mr Grey encouraged an environment where staff could talk freely about the negative and positive aspects of the client care. He supported staff members who were finding it difficult and facilitated ongoing discussion, while using his own expertise and experience to ask and answer questions. All staff views were given equal value so care assistants could feel they were truly participating in the process. The result was that, over a period of time, all the clients had up-to-date care plans that had been written by the whole team. This increased ownership of, and therefore compliance with, the plans.

1. Would this approach help you deal with any issues within your care environment?
2. What resources does your environment have to develop and support leaders and leadership approaches?

Case study 2

Mrs Hargreaves has recently taken over a residential home that has several recommendations from two previous CSCI inspections. These have not been addressed by two previous managers who had been appointed but then resigned and left in the space of six months. Mrs Hargreaves believes that the best way to get the most from her staff is to make them feel valued. Within the home there is an NVQ Level 3 qualified member of staff who appears disruptive and Mrs Hargreaves feels this may be related to the lack of a clear role for this staff member. As there is so much to do she believes that by giving him a specific project to lead on she may gain an important ally and also get the most from him by easing some of the frustration he may be feeling. As a result she decides to make him the lead for medication management within the home as this is an area where he has expressed some good ideas in the past. Through close supervision she assists him without taking over and he thrives in the role. By the time of the next inspection he is able to indicate clear signs of improvement and shows inspectors plans for ongoing training and development of colleagues in the home. This leads to the home scoring a three* in the inspection and positive comments from CSCI about the home.

1. Who are the potential leaders within your care environment?
2. What skills do managers need to have to promote an environment where leaders can develop within long-term care settings?

*See note page 46.

Activities

1. Reflect on your own position in your organisation. Are you a manager, leader or administrator or a combination of all three? (See Definitions and Theories of Leadership.)
2. How would you describe your leadership style? Do you think your subordinates would agree with you? (See Characteristics of Leadership and The 'best fit' approach.)
3. Reflect on your own organisation. Do you have any leaders? If so, do they have the characteristics of leadership? What positions do the leaders hold? What style/s of leadership do they illustrate? (See Style theories.)

Chapter 5

Team building

INTRODUCTION

The topic of team building will enable you to address National Occupational Standard C10 'Develop teams and individuals'. In this chapter you will:

- consider the different theories related to team building;
- examine the problems that can be encountered in a team;
- examine the qualities and role of the team leader;
- consider the different roles people assume in teams;
- examine the practical issues involved in building a team.

THE THEORY AND PRACTICE OF TEAM BUILDING

Much of health and social care involves working in teams. These teams include:

- teams of the same discipline, for example nursing teams;
- consultants with teams of people or 'firms' working with them;
- multidisciplinary teams, for example, those involved in the care of the elderly, with teams including nurses, social workers, physiotherapists and occupational therapists.

In many care areas, management has become less hierarchical with teams making a bigger contribution. Such teamwork is particularly relevant in times of change as everyone needs to be involved in order to manage change effectively (Stewart, 1996).

Effective managers need the skills to build up and motivate a team and a team must also be managed. A team is not just a group of people with a common aim. A team is a group of people working together in which each individual's contribution is seen as complementary to the contribution of the other team members.

I have been involved in many teams, as a member or as a leader. My earliest experience of leadership occurred when I was at school. I was made house games captain by default because I was the only person in my house in the sixth form who played games. Despite this I decided that the house was going to win the cup for games as it had not won for over 20 years. Therefore, all house members were encouraged to play for the house teams, everyone who came to practise had a chance of getting in the team, and those who did not practise would not be chosen, even if they did play for school teams. We won every game except the junior netball that year and we won the cup. The experience brought home to me the value of team playing and the power of positive motivation.

1. Think about the best team you ever worked with. What made the best team? (See also Chapter 4: Leadership.)

THE PROBLEMS OF TEAM WORKING

Team working has some inherent problems:

- Teams may be immature (i.e. they have not been working together very long), time consuming or unpredictable and therefore difficult to manage – particularly multidisciplinary teams.
- There is often confusion over the role of the team.
- It can be difficult and time-consuming to reach agreement within a team.
- In a team there is an opportunity to shape your role as you would like it but this can be a problem if no one else thinks your role should be the one you would like.
- The manager may lobby sympathetic members to get them to sell ideas to the rest of the team.

Motivation

Individual team members are likely to be motivated by different things:

- **Comfort drive** – some like financial security and are motivated by money.
- **Structure** – some team members like certainty and thrive in bureaucracies; they like to have their role clearly delineated and they can feel threatened by change.
- **Relationships** – on the other hand, some people prefer collaborative working and like to work in teams.
- **Recognition and status** – people who are motivated by recognition and status often gravitate to professional and academic work, and they respond to praise from individuals that they rate highly.

- **Power** – some people seek a degree of influence and control (for example, professionals) and gravitate if possible to the top of an organisation.
- **Autonomy** – some people like the opportunity for individual creativity and growth.

When setting up a team and trying to motivate team members, it is important to consider what motivates the individuals who make up your team. After all, their motivation may be the opposite of yours and you may feel that they cannot see sense. Or they may have the same motivation as you and you may end up competing with them for, say, recognition and status within the team.

Reflection

In times of change the individual motivation of team members can be a problem. It can lead to different team members 'not singing from the same hymn sheet'. Those who like a structured workplace may feel threatened, while those who seek power may take the opportunity to try to gain it.

1. How do you motivate yourself? How do you motivate others?
   (See Motivation and Qualities of the Team Leader.)

QUALITIES OF A TEAM LEADER

Effective team leaders usually have the following attributes:

- An awareness of the motivation of individual team members. Each person can have a different motivation. Motivation can also be influenced by professional pressures, or by peer and group pressures.
- A clear expectation of the role of the team. Expectations must be stated explicitly and should not be assumed to be implicit. Therefore, it should not be assumed that everyone knows what the team is supposed to be doing; there must be explicit agreement with team members about the team's role.
- The team leader needs to ensure that there is a realistic possibility of achieving the team's goals as this will help develop high team morale.
- The leader needs to be aware that it is easy to build a team spirit when the team is winning but it is far more necessary to have team spirit when the team is losing.
- The team leader needs to know and understand the team's expectations of their leader.

- The team leader must give constructive and positive feedback. It is common, particularly in the public services, for team members to receive only negative feedback. This leads to the assumption that if a team does not receive feedback there is not a problem.
- The leader needs to avoid 'group think'. This is when members of the team do not debate issues, but 'go along with the most vocal' in order to avoid conflict.
- The team leader must have an awareness of any informal culture.
- A leader needs to actively resolve conflicts. There can be a tendency not to confront any conflict, which can lead to feelings of frustration among team members. Conflicts should be identified early and dealt with actively and positively.
- The team leader needs to appreciate demonstrations of appropriate loyalty.
- A leader should encourage the development of mutual trust and a sense of common purpose.
- It is important to make sure ability is the key factor in decision making rather than allowing influence and position to be decisive.
- A leader should appreciate the different team members' individual learning styles.

Effective managers also need the following skills to build up and motivate a team:

- **Power** – is an ability to impose one's will or to control or influence others.
- **Authority** – is the right to use power.
- **Success** – is influenced by a leader's attributes and style of leadership. There needs to be a sense in the team that there is a realistic possibility of achieving success and this helps to develop a high team morale.

Reflection

Consider the national football team. Its role is clear – it should win matches. Each player has a defined role such as, for example, the goalkeeper who is meant to prevent the opposition from scoring a goal. The captain is the leader and the coach provides constructive feedback.

1. What is your role in your team? Do the other team members agree this is your role? (See Qualities of a Team Leader and Team Roles.)

Key Learning Points

Effective managers need the skills to build and motivate teams:

- Teams can be difficult to manage;
- Motivations of team members may differ;
- Team leaders need to have many different qualities.

TEAM ROLES

The following is a description of nine common roles people may adopt in teams. You do not have to have nine people to have a successful team, but a team will be more effective if all nine roles are covered by team members. Some members of a team may well play more than one role in the team and enjoy the variety that this brings. Other team members may have a preference for one particular role and find it difficult to fulfil more than one role at a time (Belbin 1993).

Co-ordinator (Chairman)

The co-ordinator guides the group and defines priorities, allocates tasks and roles and recognises the talent of team members, while not being threatened by them. The co-ordinator is concerned with what is feasible, rather than with what is exciting and imaginative.

Shaper

The shaper is task oriented, will push the team to achieve the task, and may take a leader role as part of the team in order to keep the group focused.

Team worker

The team worker looks after the relationships in the group and is more concerned with the process than the task, and with the welfare of the individuals in the team. A team worker tends to be perceptive of peoples' needs and adept at supporting individuals.

Plant innovators

Plant innovators are the 'ideas people'. They often originate ideas and they can be defensive, though they will be evangelical when convinced of the points of view of other team members. Their concern for good ideas can overshadow their ability to be sensitive to the needs of other team members.

Resource investigator

Resource investigators tend to trade in ideas, rather than provide them. They spot good ideas, collect information with the aim of supporting the team's efforts and put ideas together. They prompt further thinking by encouraging discussion.

Monitor/evaluator

The monitor/evaluators tend to be less enthusiastic, but more objective. They will carefully and critically analyse all the arguments.

Completer finisher

The completer finisher makes sure the group meets the deadlines and finishes the tasks. They harness all the anxiety and concern about getting the job done on time and to a high standard.

Company worker

The company worker implements the ideas and translates them into practice. They are also concerned with the practicalities and the feasibility of the processes.

Specialist

The specialist is the expert adviser who may be needed to ensure the project succeeds.

Belbin (1993) said that individuals working in a team were predisposed to have a dominant role, but may also show a tendency to take on other roles, particularly if a role is missing in a team. Usually the role taken by a team member is linked to their own reasoning abilities, motivations and personality characteristics. However, it is also influenced by the other members of the team and the roles that they play, and is affected by the priorities and processes of the team leader. Team leaders need to make an assessment of role strengths of staff, encourage flexibility and, if there are missing roles in the team, ask other members of the team to take them on, delegating if necessary, as this should improve the functioning of the team. Even if all the skills are available this does not mean that conflict is avoided, but a leader can head off tensions and avoid a group breakdown. Awareness of the role or roles of others can also assist team members to value the contributions of all members of the team.

Reflection

Joining a work team can be a fraught experience for a newcomer. Often, agency workers do not expect to be considered part of the team when they turn up for work as they will only be there for a shift. Work teams may reciprocate this attitude, which can then become self-fulfilling. The agency worker works on their own, having been asked to carry out the tasks no one else wants to do, and they then make a resolution never to return.

1. How do you deal with new or temporary members of your team?

TEAM BEHAVIOUR

Team behaviour is determined by:

- the style and personality of the leader;
- group norms of the standards of behaviour within teams (thinking about the teams to which you belong, what are regarded as the 'normal' standards of behaviour in each team and do these norms differ from team to team?);
- team cohesion (i.e. loyalty to the team);
- the roles played by members – roles are interpreted differently by individual members and some of this behaviour may well be cultural;
- the nature and motivation of its members;
- the nature of the task;
- the size of the group – in large groups some members avoid participation and it is often the case that the larger the group the less likely it is that the task will be completed;
- the environment in which the group operates.

As a manager you may inherit a team or you may become part of a team and, in the short term, you will be constrained by the size of the team, its membership, the members' knowledge and the task set. A team that is already formed will have its own motivation, methods of interacting and have a record of effectiveness. Participation is related positively to the size of a team – the larger the team the more likely members are to be absent, and the lower the morale. The optimum size for a team is five to seven members, which means that members of teams are often required to adopt more than one role (see Team Roles).

FACTORS THAT INFLUENCE TEAM WORKING

	The group	The task	The environment
The givens,	Size	Nature	Norms and expectations
	• Member characteristics; • Individual objectives; • Stage of team development.	• Criteria for effectiveness; • Importance of the task; • The clarity of the task.	• Leader position; • Inter-group relations.
… which all affect the intervening actors,		• Choice of leadership style; • Processes and procedures; • Motivation.	
…which determine the outcomes.		• Productivity, • Member satisfaction.	

Key Learning Points

Team leaders need to be aware of their team's role strengths:

- Members of teams take on different roles and some members may have more than one role;
- Team behaviours have varied determinants which the leader needs to be aware of;
- The leader needs to understand the team, the task and the environment in which they are operating.

BUILDING A TEAM

To build a team you must have clear and specific aims and objectives. These aims and objectives must be:

- measurable;
- achievable;
- realistically timed.

The time taken to develop a fully functioning team should not be underestimated. Circumstances will vary but team members have to be encouraged to build up relationships over a period of time.

> ### Reflection
>
> Think of teams you have joined. It will have taken time for you to build up a relationship with other team members. Team-building away days can help but often social occasions can be a better way for members of a team to get to know each other.
>
> 1. Think of the last team that you joined. How long did it take you to feel a member of the team? What, in particular, helped the process?

The team leader must:

- plan and monitor progress;
- take time to develop the team;
- have the necessary skills and resources;
- ensure that they have the appropriate knowledge, skills and ability available to help individuals avoid being overwhelmed by the task or team (this means that if there are any gaps in the help available the leader must try to fill them);
- recognise individual achievement and acknowledge members of staff who are more effective than the team leader;
- ensure that the team has the ability to work together and is balanced in terms of roles and motivation;
- be able to both give and receive feedback;
- be able to analyse what is happening in the team, and deal with the issues as they occur.

ISSUES RELATING TO HEALTH AND SOCIAL CARE TEAM WORKING

Much of caring is carried out as a team. However, some professions are more reliant on team working in their daily work than others. Some professionals prefer working in teams or, at the very least, with another member of staff. In part this can be because it is easier to carry out some physical tasks with two people; for example, making a bed is a lot quicker with two people. Staff members who are used to team working often prefer it and may well dislike working in isolation. It can also be much easier to build a team when everyone expects to work as a team.

Multidisciplinary teams are now more common in health and social care. The bringing together of different professionals from different work areas provides a range of expertise. However, building multidisciplinary teams may require more expertise on the part of the team leader. Different professionals will not only have different working experiences, they may also have different values, group norms and expectations of their position or role in a team than the other members of the team. To enable effective team building it is essential that both roles and lines of accountability are clarified in a multidisciplinary team.

Finally, the integration of information technology may influence the way a team works and it can also lead to the formation of 'virtual' teams. It is important to be aware that different skills are required to communicate at a distance, and that electronic communication is often less formal.

Reflection

As a goal-keeper in a hockey team, I appreciated playing with a very good back player. She was so good I never saw the ball, so we won all our games. Most of you will have had similar experiences of working well with certain team members, despite the amount of work that had to be done, as well as the experience of having a miserable shift because you were working with different team members. On one ward I worked on, a nurse finished the care of her own patients and then gave them a cup of tea and washed the teapot. Because she did not think that she was part of a team she didn't consider giving out tea to the patients of other nurses who were still busy.

1. Think of a team you have enjoyed working in. What, in particular, made the work enjoyable?

Key Learning Points

Building a team requires:

- Planning, development and time;
- Consideration of factors and issues such as information technology that may change the way your team works and communicates;
- The ability to understand how to work with different professionals in order to build effective multidisciplinary teams.

Summary of Key Learning Points

Effective managers need the skills to build and motivate teams:

- Teams can be difficult to manage;
- Motivations of team members may differ;
- Team leaders need to have many different qualities.

Team leaders need to be aware of their team's role strengths:

- Members of teams take on different roles and some members may have more than one role;
- Team behaviours have varied determinants which the leader needs to be aware of;
- The leader needs to understand the team, the task and the environment in which they are operating.

Building a team requires:

- Planning, development and time;
- Consideration of factors and issues such as information technology that may change the way your team works and communicates;
- The ability to understand how to work with different professionals in order to build effective multidisciplinary teams.

Case study 1

Gill Chambers is a new member of staff who is in her mid-forties and is coming into care work for the first time. Her previous career had been in banking where she was head of a regional team of diverse employees. She had left this career to look after her mother and, after her mother's death, Mrs Chambers decided that she wanted to work in the care field full time. She has been employed as a team leader by a manager of a home that has had problems with team working in the past. The manager feels that her skills will be valuable in addressing these problems. She places her on the busiest unit within the home, which has the most issues. Gill is not keen to accept this role as it is not why she came into this field but, because it is a way into the profession, she accepts the job. On introducing her to the unit manager the home manager makes it very clear why she has put Gill in that unit. The relationship between Gill and the unit manager is difficult from the start and members of staff clearly follow one or the other. Within a month the team on the unit seems even more divided and both the manager and Gill appear frustrated. Both have indicated that if things do not improve they are going to resign.

1. What advice would you give to the home manager in this situation?
2. What could help both Gill and the unit manager to improve the situation?
3. Which team member types would be most helpful in a situation like this?

Case study 2

Old Street is a six-bedded supported living unit for people with learning disabilities. Most of the residents have lived there for over three years. The relatives are a very vocal and active group who strongly advocate the rights of the residents. Over the last few years a confrontational relationship has developed between the relatives and the staff. Both sides effectively want the same things for the residents but can never seem to agree on how to move the unit forward. The manager has recently attended a team-building course and feels that she has some ideas on how to improve the relationships. Ideas include communicating with the relatives and her staff on how to move forward.

1. If you were the manager in this situation, what would you do to improve things?

Activities

1. How large is your team? Who do you include in your team and why? (See Theory and Practice of Team Building).
2. What are your motives when working in a team? Reflect on what you think are the motives of other members of your team. Try to check them out (tactfully). (See Motivation.)
3. Reflect on your own leadership of your team. Alternatively, if you are not yet a team leader, reflect on the team or teams you work in and your team leader(s). Do you know what your team expects from you? Compare your thoughts about your own team reflection with your thoughts about the other teams you may be part of, such as, for example, a management team. What are the differences? Asking members of your team to complete a questionnaire on their opinion of the qualities of a team leader could be a helpful activity. (See Qualities of a Team Leaders.)

4. Reflecting on your own team, what role/s does each member play? Are they effective in their roles and, if not, why not? What part do you normally play in your team? (See Team Roles.)
5. Does your team function well and, if not, why not? How could its performance be improved? (See Building a Team and Qualities of a Team Leader.)

Part 4 of Stewart (1996) could be helpful for answering some of these questions.

FURTHER READING

Stewart, R. (1996) *Leading in the NHS*. Macmillan Business.

Chapter 6

Group working

INTRODUCTION

The topic of group working will enable you to address National Occupational Standards C13 'Manage the performance of teams and individuals' and C10 'Develop teams and individuals'. In this chapter you will:

- consider the theory and practice of group working;
- identify the stages of group formation;
- be aware of the effect of groups on decision making;
- consider the effects of learning and relationship styles on groups;
- be aware of harmful effects on groups and the factors that make groups effective or ineffective;
- use checklists to analyse how your groups function;
- be aware of communication patterns in groups.

THE THEORY AND PRACTICE OF GROUP WORKING

Whenever a new member joins a team or group the dynamics of the group change and the group needs to re-establish its method of working in order to continue functioning effectively. When a new member joins a stable team the effect is often noticeable. However, in places where team members change on a daily basis with different shifts, staff members may never actually work together as a functioning team and a new group member may not have a noticeable impact.

Groups work in an environment, usually an organisation, and not in isolation. Organisations often impose unavoidable norms on groups and have expectations about the ways groups should function, and these may or may not be appropriate to the group. The physical environment in which a group functions can also influence the amount of interaction within the group. Physical barriers can prevent groups forming but poor facilities and/or isolation can actually increase group cohesion such as, for example, with coal miners.

Stages of group formation

Tuckman and Jensen (1977) indentified the stages of group formation based on Tuckman's (1965) earlier work, but added the important concept of adjourning (see Figure 1).

Forming (a group of individuals)

- Talk about the purpose of the group;
- The definition and title of the group;
- The composition of the group;
- The leadership pattern;
- The life span of the group;
- Individuals tend to want to make an impression at this stage.

Storming (the conflict stage)

- When preliminary and often false consensus on purposes is discussed;
- When leadership and other roles are decided;
- Norms of work and behaviour are challenged and re-established;
- Personal agendas are revealed;
- There can be inter-personal hostility but if successfully handled this can result in a more realistic setting of objectives, procedures and norms;
- This stage is important for testing the norms of trust in the group.

Norming. The group needs to:

- establish norms and practices;
- decide when and how it should work;
- decide how it should take decisions;
- decide on the type of behaviour expected;
- decide on the level of work;
- decide on the degree of openness;
- decide on the appropriate trust and confidence;
- allow tentative experimentation by individuals, which enables them to test the temperature of the group and measure the appropriate level of their commitment.

Performing (occurs when the previous stages have been successfully completed):

- The group reaches full maturity and is able to be fully and sensibly productive;
- The group can be productive earlier, but is likely to be impeded by personal agendas;
- The agenda and leadership are questioned.

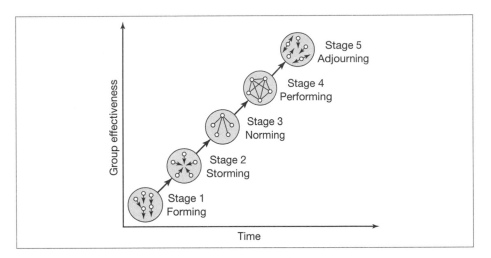

Figure 1 The stages of small group development (based on Tuckman and Jensen, 1977, 'Stages of small group development revisited', in Huczynski and Buchanan, 1991, p. 175).

Adjourning:

- The group breaks up but may form another group;
- This can happen when new members join.

Key Learning Points

Changes in groups are influenced by:

- New members;
- Changes in function or task;
- Changes over time;
- The stage the group is at.

DECISION MAKING IN GROUPS

All groups have their own style of decision making. This is often influenced by the function of the group. It is important that decisions are made in the appropriate style for that group so that it can function effectively. Decisions in a group can be taken by:

- the person in authority (autocratic);
- the majority (democratic);
- a consensus (democratic);
- a minority (can be a powerful minority);
- any member of the group who assumes that no one will object (*laissez-faire*, individual approach).

77

> ## Reflection
>
> By the end of the 1970s consensus management was common in the NHS. At the unit (hospital) level of management and above, representatives from medicine, nursing and administration were expected to make decisions together. However, the professions often had different philosophies and objectives to those of the administration. This often led to either the group members agreeing with the most forthright character or, alternatively, very little decision making actually taking place. Failing to make decisions can work for a time – either the situation will resolve itself and disappear or, after a time, the solution will become evident or a compromise is made. However, this is really decision making by default and the group may not like the solution which has evolved. Decisions have to be taken and, if they are taken without participation, group members may become resentful and reluctant to participate in the group. In the NHS the situation was changed by the introduction of general management, the appointment of general managers and then, more recently, the appointment of chief executives.
>
> 1. Examine the various groups, work or social, to which you belong. Who makes the decisions and why? (See Decision Making in Groups.)

LEARNING STYLES

The members of a group differ and will have different learning styles. They may be:

- **Activists** – try anything once:
  - o They like new experiences and change, and they learn from exchanging ideas with others.
  - o They dislike solitary learning or being told exactly what and how to do something. They do not like lectures or formal teaching.
- **Theorists**:
  - o They are analytical, objective, logical and rational. They like to know exactly what they are doing and why. They learn a lot from teaching others and like formal teaching and discussions.
  - o They learn least when told to act without being given the reasons. They dislike learning with activists.
- **Reflectors**:
  - o They like to consider all the implications, learn from listening, observing and considering and reviewing previous learning.
  - o They find it difficult to work when they cannot plan or when they have incomplete information with which to make a decision.
- **Pragmatists**:
  - o These are the experimenters – practical people who try out new ideas to find those that work. They like solving problems, learning most when ideas are immediately relevant, like simulations.
  - o They dislike theories that cannot be implemented.

Some group members may well combine different styles to learn. It is important that there are also different opportunities and learning methods available to all members.

Reflection

When teaching a practical skill the principle is to show one (i.e. demonstrate the skill), then let the student perform the skill under supervision, repeating this as often as necessary until the student is able to do the procedure on their own. The same principles apply when teaching a theoretical subject. The information should be presented in different ways because, for example, some people like to learn using pictures, while others do not find pictures useful. Some people like to use a combination of methods when they are learning.

1. Do you know how you learn? (See Learning Styles.)

RELATIONSHIP STYLES

In groups people have different relationship styles. The individual's role in a group is concerned with what that person does. The personality of the person will affect the way in which they carry out their role and the way in which they interact with other group members (Iles, 1997). Different people will have different relationship styles (see Figure 2). For example:

- **Socialisers** are:
  o enthusiastic, persuasive, motivating and creative;
  o good at starting projects.
- **Directors**:
  o make sure the things that need to be done get done;
  o they take control;
  o they make decisions.
- **Relaters**:
  o are good listeners;
  o are supportive of others;
  o they build trust;
  o their aim is to collaborate not compete;
  o are sensitive and can be bullied.
- **Thinkers/analysts**:
  o are accurate;
  o they are independent;
  o they take pride in work;
  o they cannot be hurried;
  o they are critical of mistakes;
  o they hate surprises.

79

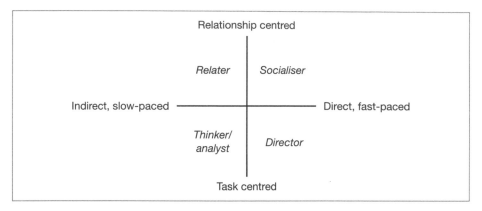

Figure 2 Relationship styles (from Iles, 1997, p. 16)

If you are putting a group together for a specific task, you need to consider the personality of the group members as well as their knowledge and skills (Stewart, 1996). It is essential that you understand the differences in personalities. Differences can cause conflict, but remember that conflict can also be made constructive and creative (Iles, 1997).

Reflection

Curriculum planning is a common task in health and social care education. A group starts with a blank piece of paper and ends up with a lengthy document. To achieve the end result it is important to put together a team of people that has the knowledge and the relevant up-to-date expertise in the subject. They also need to have the skills to put their ideas in writing, to work together as a team and they must be willing to share their work without being defensive. Their personalities have to be taken into account if the group is to be successful with students wanting to do the course.

1. You have been asked to design a training course for care assistants. Which colleagues would you wish to join your planning group and why? (See Relationship Styles.)

GROUP BEHAVIOUR

Behaviour between different groups

Behaviour between groups is as important as behaviour within groups (Hardy, 2005). The influence of a group and its individual members will influence the interaction between groups (Handy, 1999). Competition between groups can either be harmful or have a useful effect on the groups.

Harmful effects

- Groups can develop conflicting goals.
- Groups lose the ability to communicate and co-operate with each other.
- Tribalism and stereotyping of others develops.

Useful effects

- Groups develop strong cohesiveness (loyalty) among their own members.
- They develop a high regard for their task.
- There is a need to reward for contribution to the common good.
- There is a need to encourage communication and co-operation within the group in order to avoid win-lose situations.

Behaviour within groups

Effective groups	Ineffective groups
Informal, relaxed atmosphere.	Bored or tense atmosphere.
Much relevant discussion with a high degree of participation.	Discussion dominated by one or two people, and often irrelevant.
Group task or objective clearly understood and commitment to it obtained from group members.	No clear common objective.
Members listen to one another.	Members tend not to listen to each other.
Conflict is not avoided, but dealt with openly and constructively.	Conflict is either avoided or allowed to develop into open warfare.
Most decisions are reached by a general consensus with a minimum of voting.	Simple majorities are seen as sufficient basis for group decisions, which the minority have to accept.
Ideas are expressed freely and openly.	Personal feelings are kept hidden and criticism is embarrassing.
Leadership is not always with the chair, but tends to be shared as appropriate.	Leadership is provided by the chair.
The group examines its own progress and behaviour.	The group avoids any discussion about its own behaviour.

Key Learning Points

The way a group functions may be influenced by:

- Different learning styles in the group;
- Different relationship styles;
- Behaviours within the group.

ANALYSING GROUPS

An in-depth analysis will help to clarify how the group or team functions. Using your team or group as an example, work through the following checklists and analyse the results. Completing this detailed analysis may help to move a 'stuck' group forward.

Background

1. What is the group's story so far? When did the group come into being and for what purpose?
2. Has the purpose of the group changed? If so, when did this occur and why?
3. What is the composition of the group? What is the previous experience and personal history of each member? How were they related?
4. What are the key experiences of success and failure which the group shares?
5. What expectations does each member have of the group and of their role in it?

Team

1. Is the size and make-up of the team correct? Should a sub-team be set up?
2. Are opportunities and/or procedures in place to ensure everyone participates in decision making?
3. Do you restructure and change individuals' jobs as appropriate?

Participation patterns

1. How much of the talking is done by the leader and how much is done by the other members?
2. To whom are questions usually addressed – the group as a whole, the leader, or particular members?

3. Do the members who don't talk much appear to be interested and listening alertly (non-verbal participation), or do they seem bored and apathetic?
4. Do the leader and other senior members in the group practise gate-keeping skills, i.e. do they open the door to allow lower-status members to talk? Draw up a picture of your group's participation patterns at your next meeting (see Figure 3).

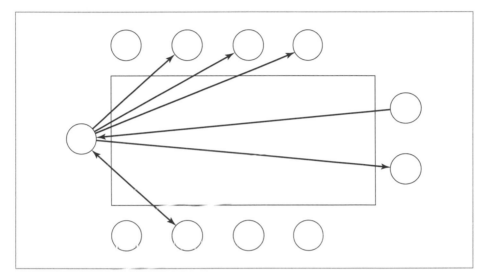

Figure 3 Group participation patterns

Group participation patterns are important as they can be very revealing about management style and about how the organisation works as a whole. In the example in Figure 3 almost all the communication is one way. The meeting is being run in an authoritative way with little participation from the group as a whole. Some members of the group are silent throughout.

How to draw a participation pattern

Start with a simple drawing of the table used and circles indicating the number and position of participants (see Figure 4). Note that if you use a round table or no table at all, make sure you reproduce this as it affects the communication pattern. A volunteer from the group should draw an arrow every time a member of the group speaks, indicating to whom they spoke and who replied to whom. For example, comments with a response should be indicated with a double-headed arrow and comments without a response should be indicated with a single arrow (see Figure 3). A few pointers:

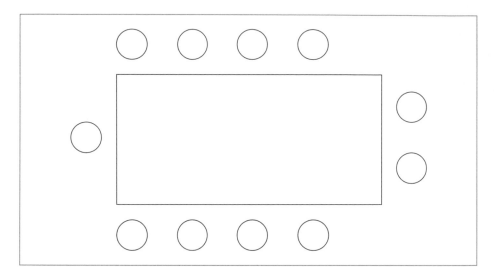

Figure 4 A template for drawing group participation patterns

1. The group should decide if the volunteer should be a participant or non-participant observer – that is, should they take their normal role in the group or just watch?
2. To record the interactions of a full meeting would be very complex. It is probably better to 'sample' a five- or ten-minute segment at the mid-point of the meeting, and not at the beginning or end of the meeting as at these points interactions tend to be different.
3. The whole exercise can be anonymous or participants identified for training purposes.

Experiments to demonstrate communication patterns have shown the following common features (see Figure 5):

• The web or authoritarian group is the quickest to make decisions as the person at the centre of the web determines the outcome.
• The ladder or bureaucratic group, where there is an inflexible hierarchy, is the slowest to make decisions.
• If the problem is complex, the all-channel or networking group is likely to produce the best solution. These are democratic groups.
• For an individual, satisfaction is highest if they are at the centre of the web, followed by individuals in the all-channel or networking group. The ladder is the lowest in terms of satisfaction overall, but the people on the periphery of the web can feel very isolated.

Use of the group participation pattern diagram (Figures 3 and 4) will help to diagnose your group's participation pattern.

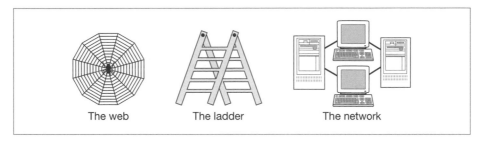

The web   The ladder   The network

Figure 5 Examples of communication patterns (based on Handy, 1986 and 1999)

Communication

1. Are members expressing their ideas clearly, simply and concisely?
2. Are visual aids and other communication aids used in a way that suggests thorough preparation by members?
3. Do any general concepts such as, for example, 'maximum profit' or 'customer service' get sufficiently defined so that the group agrees on their meaning?
4. Do members often adopt contributions previously made and build their ideas on to them?
5. Do members feel free to ask for clarification when they don't understand a statement?
6. Are responses to statements frequently irrelevant?

Cohesiveness

1. How well is the group working together as a unit?
2. What sub-groups or 'lone wolves' are there and how do they affect the group?
3. What evidence is there of interest or lack of interest on the part of members of the group (or groups in the organisation) in what is happening in the area of the common task?
4. Do members speak to the leader of 'your group' or 'our group'?
5. Despite reverses, is the level of confidence high? Is there still a strong sense of purpose and resolve?
6. Is the team spirit in evidence? Do members mutually support and encourage each other as well as working well together in a technical sense?

Atmosphere

1. Would you describe your primary work group as warm or cool, friendly or hostile, relaxed or tense, informal or formal, free or restrained?
2. Can opposing views or negative feelings be expressed without fear of retribution?
3. Is morale in the group low? Is there an 'atmosphere of doubt, of looking back'?

Key Learning Points

Group patterns can be analysed by examining:

- Background, the team, participation patterns, communication, cohesiveness and atmosphere;
- Research on communications in groups.

Summary of Key Learning Points

Changes in groups are influenced by:

- New members;
- Changes in function or task;
- Changes over time;.
- The stage the group is at.

The way a group functions may be influenced by:

- Different learning styles in the group;
- Different relationship styles;
- Behaviours within the group.

Group patterns can be analysed by examining:

- Background, the team, participation patterns, communication, cohesiveness and atmosphere;
- Research on communications in groups.

Case study 1

Wall Street is a care home for people with dementia. The home has four residential units and one unit providing Category 1 NHS care. The unit was transferred from a local hospital that was in the process of closing down. The staff team, although now being employed within a private sector environment, are mainly NHS employees transferred with the unit. To cover vacancies, staff provided by the home were transferred into the unit and the unit was to be directly managed by the home manager. Staff and relatives had expressed concern about the transfer and had made it clear that they were dubious about the ability of a care home to meet the needs of the clients. Within six months one of the non-NHS staff had been reported by the relatives for bad practice and this was supported by the unit manager and another NHS care assistant. Complaints were raised by staff about the quality of the support given by the home. Three of the staff nurses arranged a meeting with a union representative to complain about the management style of the home manager and insisted on transfer back to alternative NHS settings. Relatives of clients recently transferred to the unit complained of feeling pressured by some of those who had been part of the transfer to complain about care. Although they were more positive about the environment and some of the care being delivered, they were concerned about the atmosphere within the unit. They also felt that any issues they tried to discuss with certain staff would be used against them. New staff complained of feeling excluded and victimised.

The home manager discussed these problems in supervision with her line manager with a view to identifying underlying issues and to work on a plan to start to repair the unit. She felt that she had to be realistic about people's feelings regarding the transfer but, at the same time, get the unit to the appropriate level while not compromising herself, her staff or her residents.

1. What dynamics are at play in this situation?
2. What stage of development is this team at?
3. How can the manager start to address the problems on the unit?

Case study 2

Mr Jake is the deputy manager of a small home split into two ten-bedded units. The home has a good reputation within the local community and has received several good inspection reports. The only requirement of the last inspection is that the workforce needs to reflect the ethnic and cultural make-up of the client group. The home is situated within an urban area with a multicultural population. However, the client group is mainly of white European background. They are an eloquent group who have expressed willingness to be involved in the on-going development of the home, so Mr Jake decides to discuss how he might meet this requirement with them. He is concerned that this may lead to some potential issues regarding the race of his current employees but feels that even if this happens it may be better to have an honest discussion about it. The senior carer is African and comes to see him with concerns from staff that this meeting may compromise the employment of some of the staff. Mr Jake is able to confirm that this will not happen. The senior carer says that she would like to be part of the meeting so that she can then deal with any concerns raised. The meeting is very well attended and is facilitated by Mr Jake and a resident who had a career in business management. From the meeting the following points arise:

- The residents stated that they were not concerned about where people came from as long as the staff worked in a way that fitted in with the culture of the home.
- Residents did have issues with language barriers but had not felt comfortable in raising this through fear of being labelled as racist.
- Residents stated that the best way for ensuring new staff matched their needs was for them to be involved in the recruitment process.

To address the issues raised the following action points were developed:

- Three of the residents would be given training on the home's equal opportunities and recruitment programmes, and would then sit on interview panels.
- A regular staff and resident forum would be held where all parties could discuss concerns about the home in an honest and open way.
- One resident who had been a teacher for students who did not have English as a first language would offer teaching and support to staff who requested this.

Copies of the notes from the meeting were sent to the local CSCI department, which then commended the home on its approach.

1. Which stage of group formation is this team at?
2. Are the residents/patients within your working environment part of the team?
3. If yes, how can you best use their skills, knowledge and experience?
4. If no, is this something you would like to achieve and how are you going to do this?

Activities

1. Reflect on your own group. Is it working as a group? If not, what stage is the group at? Why do you feel it is at this stage? (See Stages of group formation.)
2. How are decisions taken in your group? Does the process work well? If so, why? If not, why not? (See Decision Making in Groups.)
3. Reflect on the way you prefer to learn. What methods do you use if you are trying to impart information to a group? Do you have difficulties getting messages across? (See Learning Styles.)
4. Draw up a group participation pattern for a group you attend regularly. (See Participation patterns.)
5. Think about your own behaviour in a group. What type of relationship style do you exhibit? Can you identify which of the other styles are present? Again, people do not necessarily exhibit only one style and, of course, their style can change depending on the styles of other members of the group, and on the type of group. (See Relationship Styles.)

Chapter 7

Appraisal

INTRODUCTION

The topic of appraisal will enable you to address National Occupational Standards C10 'Develop teams and individuals' and C13 'Manage the performance of teams and individuals'. In this chapter you will:

- consider definitions and theories of appraisal;
- identify the purpose of appraisal;
- examine the problems and hazards of appraisal;
- assess different methods of performance measurement;
- consider the appraiser's need for objectivity and training;
- assess your own appraisal skills.

DEFINITIONS AND THEORIES OF APPRAISAL

Appraisal is an evaluation of the performance or potential performance of employees. It is not a new innovation:

> The imperial rater seldom rates according to the merits of the individual but always rates according to his likes and dislikes.
>
> China 1,700 years ago

Since the introduction of general management in health and social care, there has been more emphasis on performance appraisal. For example, Agenda for Change, a method of assessing pay using performance reviews, has recently been introduced into the NHS. Employment legislation has also played a part because it is important to have documentation of an employee's performance and the help they have received if you ever need to apply disciplinary procedures. Different names are given to the appraisal process depending on the organisation, such as: staff assessment; employee review; staff reporting; performance review; performance evaluation. However, the general principles should be the same.

Appraisal is one of the few times that an employee is evaluated as an individual as, for much of the time, employees are viewed as being part of a team or group. There are two main types of appraisal: formal and informal. Informal appraisal is carried out day-to-day, particularly if you work alongside or in a group with the staff you have to appraise. Formal appraisal is rational, orderly, documented and normally done once a year with, perhaps, a follow-up at intervals throughout the year.

THE OBJECTIVES OF APPRAISAL

Management information

The appraisal process can provide the following management information:

- Existing and potential manpower strengths and weaknesses.
- As the basis for determining rewards, transfers, redundancies and dismissals (some appraisal policies specifically exclude the above: always check your organisation's policy before performing appraisals and/or before being appraised).
- Determining training needs.
- Identifying criteria against which to measure performance.
- Evaluating existing performance.
- Enabling an employee to improve their performance.
- Succession planning.

Motivation

The appraisal process can help to provide staff motivation by:

- identifying strengths and weaknesses, and by providing feedback;
- helping to plan personal and job objectives and identifying ways to achieve these;
- helping to improve performance.

Assessment of potential

You can use the appraisal process to assess staff potential.

- It is never reliable to look just at past performance as there may have been mitigating circumstances.
- Present performance may also not be reliable due to circumstances.
- It is often better to have your own superior involved in the assessment of potential as this can give the process more objectivity, especially when there have been problems with performance.
- Assessment centres can be used to help to assess potential, although this can be expensive. However, assessment centres will predict future performance in specific roles and they can produce a better forecast than managers as they can be more objective.

It is important to note that you should not attempt to use one appraisal meeting with a member of staff and one appraisal form to try to achieve all these objectives. You will need to measure different objectives at different times and at different stages in an individual's employment.

Reflection

How often have you been encouraged to improve your qualifications or increase your experience in an appraisal? I was interviewing a chief executive who wanted to encourage equal opportunities in his Community Trust. All jobs were advertised on a central notice board and all staff members were encouraged to apply. If they did not have the necessary qualifications or experience at the time of their application they were given feedback and help to enable them to apply for a similar job in the future.

1. Do you think appraisal is a good tool for staff development? Has this been your experience of appraisal? (See The Objectives of Appraisal.)

Performance management

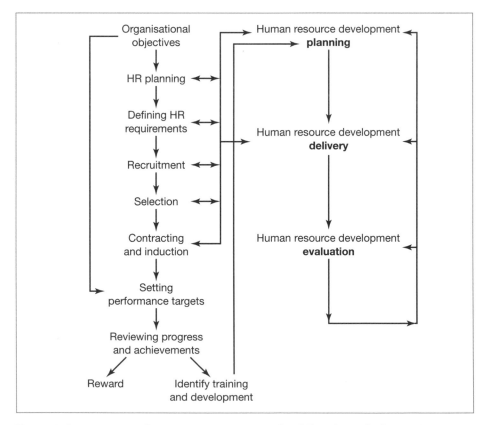

Figure 1 Integrating performance management (Blundell and Murdoch, 1997)

As can be seen in Figure 1, appraisal should fit in with an organisation's human resources policy. Of course, employees also have a responsibility for their own development and appraisals can provide them with the feedback they need to help them to do this.

> ## Reflection
>
> In nursing, if you are a good student you become a staff nurse, although this is a very different job to the one you did as a student. If you are a competent staff nurse you are promoted up the levels. The competencies expected in each level are different, so there is no guarantee that if you are good as a staff nurse you will also be good as a ward manager. However, this is the usual route for promotion for nursing staff.
>
> 1. How can appraisal help to ensure promotions are appropriate and timely? (See The Objectives of Appraisal and Performance Management.)

THE APPRAISAL PROCESS

The basic process

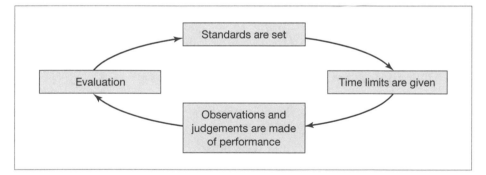

Figure 2 The four parts of performance appraisal

In an organisation there should be a standard process for appraisal interviews (see Figure 2). Guidance notes should be produced for both the appraisers and the appraisees and both parties should have a copy of the appraisal form that will be used. There are many different appraisal formats, from structured to very open appraisals, but all should contain the following elements.

1. A review of the past year based on the achievement (or not) of agreed objectives.
2. Discussion of the key issues affecting the non-achievement of objectives.
3. Discussion of the year ahead including activities, responsibilities and setting new objectives where appropriate.
4. Discussion of any training and development needed to help where objectives were not achieved and any additional training or support that is needed to fulfil the coming year's objectives.

Elements 1 and 2 are the responsibility of the appraisee and 3 and 4 are the responsibility of the appraiser, although all elements should be subject to mutual discussion.

ACAS (Advisory, Conciliation and Arbitration Service) provides useful advice on appraisal and some sample formats that are free of copyright and can be adapted for your own use. Formats are available on the ACAS website: **www.acas.org.uk/index.aspx?articleid=651**.

MEASURING PERFORMANCE

An employee's performance can be categorised in the following ways:

- If they don't understand cooking then this would be a managerial problem and training may be required.
- If they can't cook then this would be a capability problem and they may be in the wrong job, or training may be required.
- If they won't cook despite knowledge of cooking, then this is a disciplinary problem.

There are various methods of measuring performance objectively. Two common methods are using rating scales and setting objectives. Both of these methods have strengths and weaknesses.

Using rating scales

Behaviourally anchored rating scale
- These scales identify important behaviours like, for example, communication, teamwork and effectiveness in the role (which includes the quality of their work – see Figure 3).
- Staff should participate in defining the important dimensions of the scale as they usually have the most knowledge of their job.

Quality of work – tick appropriate box below:

Exceptional

Above average

Average

Below average

Poor

Figure 3 A behavioural scale

- The scale should describe and give examples of the required behaviour on a scale that rates behaviour from excellent through acceptable to poor.
- The scale should reduce subjectivity and will provide discussion points to use when counselling staff.
- Such scales can help the appraiser to feel more confident when tackling behavioural issues.

Problems

- Behavioural scales are time-consuming to develop.
- They can result in numerous scales and appraisal forms for different jobs in the same organisation.
- Research shows that there is actually little increase in objectivity.
- The scales measure behaviour but offer no assistance in changing behaviour.

Using linear scales

- The factors selected for the scale must be relevant and measurable (see Figure 4).

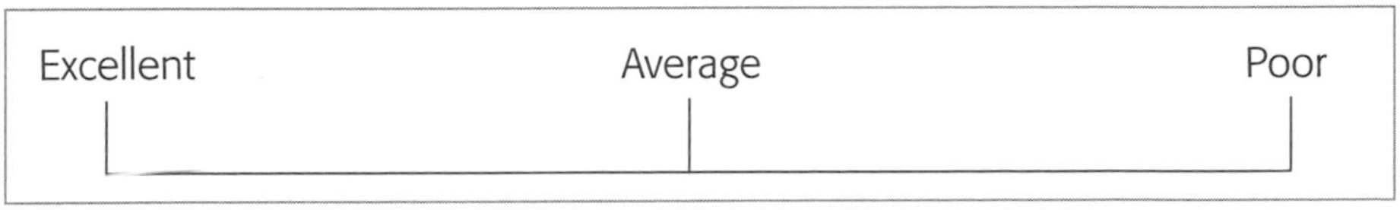

Excellent   Average   Poor

Figure 4 A linear scale

- However, the behavioural factors or traits are likely to be subjective unless they are very clearly delineated.
- Linear scales can result in greater objectivity.
- It is essential that the ability to do the job and the quality of performance required are included in the scale.

Problems

- Scales can be subjective.
- No explanation need be given for the ratings used.
- There are difficulties in measuring personal qualities.
- Such scales need to be relevant to the job and person.

Activities

1. Look at the two scales in Figures 3 and 4. What are the specific problems with these scales? Think particularly about the definitions of the words used. Do you understand exactly what is meant by these words in the context of appraisal?

Setting objectives

- Management By Objectives (MBO) is results-oriented.
- Objectives are set at one appraisal and at the following interview, progress is measured against the objectives set.
- Often the objectives set are linked to organisational goals and objectives.
- Employees can participate in setting their own objectives, which can then be used as a basis for the appraisal.
- It is important to be realistic about what can be achieved and limit the number of objectives set.

Problems with objectives

- It is difficult to compare employees regarding promotion and salary if you use an objectives-based appraisal system.
- The achievement of objectives can be dependent on the performance of others.
- Objectives are often difficult to define and are rarely consistent over a long period of time.
- Using objectives needs constant and consistent management to produce results.
- There can be an over-emphasis on organisational objectives to the detriment of personal development.

PROBLEMS OF APPRAISAL

As long as performance procedure is fair, is consistent, and is evenly applied to all, the performance appraisal is a just device that can be morally justified.

(Banner and Cooke, 1984)

It is important to be aware of the potential problems and pitfalls of appraisal. Two key problems are a) the difficulty in maintaining objectivity and b) the attitude of the appraiser (such as, for example, the attitude of the Imperial Rater in the quote at the start of this chapter). It is usual for the appraiser to be the immediate superior of the appraisee. However, a performance review can be done by 'grandparents' (i.e. the manager's own line manager), colleagues, subordinates, or the staff member and a manager (55 per cent of organisations use self-appraisal together with appraisal by an immediate superior). While it is argued that colleagues and subordinates may provide the most accurate appraisal of performance, there is no definitive proof that this is the case. Managers will also have different objectives to those of a worker's peers when they undertake an appraisal. 'Grandparents' are often included in an appraisal system in an attempt to ensure managerial objectivity.

Factors influencing appraisal

Difficulties in fairness and accuracy can be due to:

- the type of documents used;
- the style in which the appraisal is conducted;
- the culture of the organisation and the system of appraisal that it imposes on managers;
- the way the interview is conducted.

Potential problems for the appraiser

We are all human and it is very difficult to be totally objective. Not every manager is going to like every employee and vice versa. However, it is important in the interests of objectivity that the more obvious problems are avoided or the appraisal system may fall into disrepute. What follows are some of the common problems with staff appraisal.

The 'halo' effect

A person can be thought to be good and is therefore judged to be good.

Too much and too little praise

Some appraisers never give praise and others are lavish in their positive feedback. It can also be disheartening to be 'damned by faint praise'. This can be a cultural failing. For example, people in the UK tend to be less lavish with praise than the Americans.

Middle of the road appraisals

No one appears to shine or perform badly in a unit. While this may actually be the case, it is also an easy way out of not having to confront problems and/or to avoid having to acknowledge that staff could perhaps seek promotion.

Recency

What happened most recently regarding an employee's performance colours the whole year's performance. For instance, if there was a problem last week, the person is criticised in their appraisal without their previous good performance being taken into account. It can also work the other way – if you are aware that an appraisal is about to take place you can find ways to improve your performance.

Weighting

Undue weight is given to one aspect of performance. For example, if a staff member fails to start work on time, this is considered more important than their pleasant approach with patients and their reluctance to leave work before all the care has been given.

She is similar to me

There is a tendency to like people who have similar attributes to your own. However, this should not mean that these employees are praised unduly.

Staff will also consciously or unconsciously pick up your mannerisms and it is important that you are aware of this tendency.

Bias

No-one likes everyone, but personal dislikes should never influence an appraisal and it is important to be objective and fair with everyone. If it is difficult to be objective, due to circumstances, then to avoid bias another person should complete the appraisal. It is particularly important to avoid bias on the grounds of gender, race, religion, age and personality traits.

It should be remembered that poor performance may sometimes be outside the control of a staff member. For example, the staff member may be performing poorly because they have had a personal bereavement or, alternatively, if the area in which they work was short staffed and their objectives could not be achieved because of this.

Reflection

I was talking to another ward sister one night after I had come off duty. I worked in A&E and she worked in a medical ward to which we had admitted a patient during the evening. When patients were sent to wards they were accompanied by student nurses, who had to give the person in charge of the ward a report on the patient's condition. To ensure that the student had the information correct (and as part of their learning) it was practice for the student to give the A&E sister a report before the patient was transferred. The medical ward sister's comment was, 'I knew you were on duty this evening as the student gave the patient report the same way as you do.' Obviously the student had realised she would get praise from me if she copied me, and I had been unaware of this inclination.

1. How can you ensure you do not allow this tendency to influence your judgement? (See also She is similar to me.)

Inflating and reducing performance ratings

Managers tend to operate in environments where, in order for them to survive, there is an emphasis on getting results and minimising conflicts with staff. Because of this, there can be a tendency to over-inflate performance results. This can produce the following outcomes:

- It can be unfair on both poor and outstanding performers because, when accurate ratings are later given, staff members can be very disappointed.

- Over-inflation of results increases employees' eligibility for rewards but this can lead to unreal expectations, particularly if the firm does not actually perform well.
- Inflating results means the appraiser can avoid giving a poor rating on an appraisee's written record, which can be a problem if the employee is in fact underperforming and disciplinary issues subsequently arise.
- If a normally good employee has underperformed, inflating results can protect them, which can be an advantage if the problem is a temporary one.
- Appraisal records that show employees are putting in some effort, even if they are not getting results, can help with motivation.
- Inflating results means that the appraiser avoids confrontation with the appraisee, which may lead to problems later when inherent difficulties can no longer be overlooked.
- Inflating results can be used to promote a poorly performing or disliked employee, to the disadvantage both of the subsequent manager and, perhaps, the employee who may find they are 'out of their depth' in a new post.

Of course, some managers may tend to lower results in order to:

- 'Scare' a better performance from an employee. If the employee is capable of an improved performance this could be a useful tactic. However, it can lead to resentment when the employee is aware of the ploy.
- Punish difficult or rebellious staff. This can lead to problems and staff can become even more difficult if they realise there has been a personal bias.
- Encourage a problem employee to leave. However, this could backfire as an employee may find it difficult to get another job with a poor reference.
- Create a strong record which can justify disciplinary action. Again this could cause problems for the manager at a later date when they are called upon to justify their reasons for disciplining the staff member.
- Minimise the amount of rewards earned, which, again, can cause resentment.
- Comply with an organisational edict to limit high ratings, particularly when high ratings influence pay grades.

Dealing with poor performance

It is important when dealing with poor performance that certain factors should be taken into account:

- All staff may have performed poorly for some reason.
- Performance expectations were not made explicit.
- The employee was under stress.
- The employee may not be capable (physically or mentally) of doing the job.
- The employee may not have had the right training.

- There can also be a tendency to promote people beyond their competence level.

Key Learning Points

Appraisers need to be aware of:

- The objectives of appraisal;
- The possible problems of appraisal;
- The appraiser's need to be objective;
- Issues relating to poor performance.

TRAINING FOR APPRAISAL

Training in appraisal technique is essential. An appraiser should:

- have good interviewing skills;
- an ability to listen;
- be familiar with the paperwork;
- not have too many staff to appraise at any one time.

It is usual in large organisations to have specific training for those who have to undertake appraisals. In smaller organisations there may be fewer opportunities for such training but, if this is the case, it is important either to observe experienced appraisers and/or try to make the system as objective as possible by, for instance, using grandparents as well as line managers. Performance appraisal improves if:

- specific achievable goals are set and agreed with the employee – it is easy to measure clearly defined objectives;
- the manager is regarded as being helpful, facilitative and receptive to ideas;
- if praise is immediate when performance is good or when a project is completed;
- unexpected praise is also helpful;
- evaluation of performance is done at appraisal, prior to further goal setting.

(Skinner, 1972)

Total (360°) appraisal

In some organisations 360-degree appraisal is used, with feedback also provided by peers and clients as well as managers. This type of appraisal can be helpful in assisting improvement, but can take a lot longer to complete.

Alternatives to appraisal

There are other ways of providing feedback and candidates can be identified for promotion by other means. For example:

- by carrying out special assignments;
- using secondments – lateral moves;
- creating project teams and assessing performance while carrying out a specific time-limited task;
- using assessment centres.

Key Learning Points

Training can raise the appraiser's awareness of:

- The hazards of appraisal;
- Different ways of measuring performance;
- The factors that influence appraisal;
- Alternatives to appraisal.

APPRAISAL INTERVIEW STYLES

The manager tells

This is the authoritarian approach to appraisal interviews. It is not really an interview but instruction giving. Participation by the subordinate is neither wanted nor required.

The manager tells and sells

This style is still on the authoritarian side of the spectrum but the manager wishes to persuade the subordinate to do something they may not wish to do.

The manager tells and listens

With this style the manager still has an agenda but is willing to listen and accept the subordinate's point of view.

The manager shares

This is a truly interactive approach to interviewing. The subordinate is encouraged to take a full part in the interaction.

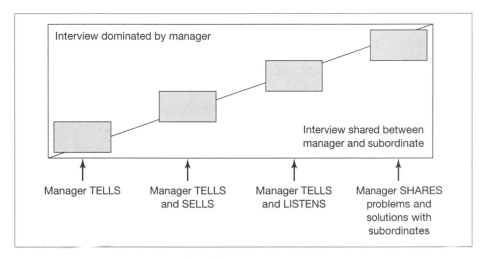

Figure 5 Appraisal interview styles (Cole, 1990, p. 435)

Reflection

A group of care assistants were discussing their upcoming appraisals. The manager and three assistant managers were going to be conducting the interviews.

Mary said: 'I hope I get Jean. She really listens but she is also good at helping me plan my year's objectives.'

Anne said: 'I like Martha. We decide my objectives together and I get to have my say.'

Jane said: 'It may seem odd but I quite like Sarah's style. She just tells me what I am doing, it's a very short interview and I know where I am.'

Sally said gloomily: 'I bet I get May. She always tries to talk me into doing things I don't really want to do.'

Of the above interviews, two were going to be appraisals and two were going to be work planning interviews. What is the difference between the two types of interview? (See The Objectives of Appraisal and Appraisal Interview Styles.)

> **Activity**
>
> Using Figure 5, reflect on the last appraisal in which you participated. If you were the manager, evaluate your performance in the process using the questions below. If you were being appraised, where did your manager come on the interview style scale?
> a. Did you praise the employee's strengths?
> b. Did you listen to their comments?
> c. Did you both agree on the goals?
> d. Can you justify the rational choices that were made?
> e. Did you constructively confront any underperformance?
> f. Had there been major changes since the last appraisals had been done?
> g. Was your staff member still feeling committed? If not, why not?
> h. Were you prepared to spend the necessary uninterrupted time with your staff?
> i. Did you ensure that the employee got something positive out of the process?
> j. Had your employee fulfilled their objectives?
> k. Did you give feedback at regular intervals?
> l. Did you allow sufficient time for the interview?

THE STAFF VIEW OF APPRAISAL

Many members of staff dislike appraisals and can be defensive about the process. The following points should always be taken into account.

- Individuals dislike admitting to any deficiencies, particularly if this could be used to control them in some way.
- The British can find it difficult to praise themselves. Other cultures may also find self-praise a problem.
- The staff member's previous relationship with the appraiser may play a part in the interview, particularly if there have been problems.
- Success is accepted as being the result of one's own efforts. Failure happens because of outside factors.
- Staff expectations of their role may not be the same as the manager's expectations. You should ensure that both parties understand what is required.
- The staff member may have seen the poor performance of other colleagues not dealt with.
- Staff may have been victims of poor managers and unrealistic expectations in the past.
- Objectives should always be measurable and achievable.
- Managers may be inadequately prepared for appraisals.
- Inadequate follow-up and lack of help to resolve problems can cause resentment.
- Problems can result if appraisals are not seen by staff to improve individual performance.

Key Learning Points

Appraisers need to be aware of:

- The continuum of interview styles;
- Their own interview style;
- Their organisation's human resources policy;
- The ways in which their staff view appraisal.

Summary of Key Learning Points

Appraisers need to be aware of:

- The objectives of appraisal;
- The possible problems of appraisal;
- The appraiser's need to be objective;
- Issues relating to poor performance.

Training can raise the appraiser's awareness of:

- The hazards of appraisal;
- Different ways of measuring performance;
- The factors that influence appraisal;
- Alternatives to appraisal.

Appraisers need to be aware of:

- The continuum of interview styles;
- Their own interview style;
- Their organisation's human resources policy;
- The ways in which their staff view appraisal.

CASE STUDIES

Appraisals make up an important part of the professional development of staff within the long-term care settings. Within the registered care home setting managers need to ensure that supervision is carried out at least six times a year. These supervision meetings can be used as a way of monitoring the progress of staff action plans as part of their annual appraisal programme.

Appraisals are often approached from one of two directions. At best they provide an opportunity for staff to express their own development needs, which the manager can then support to the benefit of the individual and the home. At worst they can be used as a management tool to address the concerns of the manager. Below are two examples of how appraisals can be used within the long-term setting.

Case study 1

Mr Harris is a qualified nurse who has studied basic psychology as part of his own professional development. In line with recommendations from the Nursing and Midwifery Council he wants to encourage an environment in which his qualified nurses have time to reflect on practice and then use experiential learning. This was discussed with all the trained staff, they were given literature on the Johns Model of Reflection (1995) and it was agreed that this would be used for both the yearly appraisal and six supervision sessions.

At the first appraisal meeting the model was discussed again. Staff members were asked to consider their own strengths and weaknesses and their own professional development – 'where would they like to be professionally in a year's time?'. It was agreed that the topics discussed in the appraisals would be the areas that the staff members focused on when writing their reflective notes. For the supervision meetings staff were encouraged to write reflective accounts of clinical incidents. These would then be discussed in detail, the positives and negatives would be removed and action plans would be developed that included training and development needs.

Over the following year the staff had developed a reflective diary and the manager had been able to link concerns about individual practice issues to the discussions in the diary so that topics were addressed in an open and constructive way. By the end of the year the manager had a much better picture of the individual strengths within the team and could allocate roles appropriately. The staff also had a reflective document that they could put into their professional portfolios. Staff found this a positive way of using the appraisal and supervision sessions, which they had previously seen as just a paper exercise.

1. What do you think about linking appraisal and supervision in this way?
2. Are there any possible problems with this approach?

Case study 2

Joan Roberts was a senior care assistant working within a small residential care home and she had been asked to take over the supervision sessions of a group of six other carers. Joan had received training in supervision but had no experience of carrying out annual appraisals. As a result she used each session as a stand-alone session. This led to each session concentrating on issues which were pertinent to the home at that particular time. Although this meant that specific needs of the home were being met, staff felt this was not addressing their personal development needs. This resulted in staff trying to use different ways to express their needs. Often this meant that they went to see their manager about working practices that could have been dealt with locally. Also, staff felt that they did not have an opportunity to continue their learning in a way that met their own needs, so some of the staff started taking courses outside of the home. Although this meant they were developing professionally they did not feel any gratitude to the home for their training and two staff, who had completed NVQ Level 2, left the home for a larger home in the area.

1. How can Joan rectify this situation?

Activities

1. What type of appraisal system is used in your work place? How often are you appraised? Is the appraisal carried out at regular intervals? Is there any follow-up between appraisals? How often are you expected to carry out appraisals? (See Definitions and Theories of Appraisal.)
2. Do you have a main objective when you carry out or participate in an appraisal? Or do you feel that appraising staff or participating in an appraisal is just a management exercise? (See The Objectives of Appraisal.)
3. Who participates in your appraisal? Do you feel it is an objective system? If not, why not? (See Problems of Appraisal.)
4. Do you normally enjoy having an appraisal? Do you get any constructive feedback between appraisals? Do you get any praise between appraisals? (See Problems of Appraisal.)
5. You have been asked to join a working party to design a new appraisal form. What would you include in the form and why? (See The Appraisal Process.)
6. You have probably had to write objectives before. What are the problems associated with setting them? Do you use a form of Management By Objectives (MBO) at work? Is it effective and, if it isn't, why isn't it? (See Measuring Performance.)

Part Two

Managing the Workplace

Chapter 8

The recruitment and selection of staff

INTRODUCTION

The topic of recruitment and selection of staff, along with other topics in Part Two, will enable you to address National Occupational Standard A1 'Assess candidates' performance'. In this chapter you will:

- learn about the principles of recruitment and selection of staff;
- address the issues involved in managing human resources;
- learn how to develop a person specification and job analysis;
- gain an understanding of the principles and practices of marketing;
- gain an understanding of the processes of shortlisting, interviewing and selecting staff.

MANAGING HUMAN RESOURCES

The organisation's human resources are its most valuable asset. If managed correctly and flexibly, staff can be part of an organisation far longer than any other resource and they can also provide 'intelligence capital'. In service industries, staff costs can be both the biggest expense and the most essential resource. Seventy-five per cent of NHS and social sector costs are estimated to be staffing and, of these staff, nursing/care workers have the largest budget. In any care setting the costs of the staff are considerable, especially if 24-hour care is provided throughout the year.

During the last 40 years there have been pressures on staffing in the care sector. The majority of health and care sector workers are typically female and their wages are low. As employment and educational opportunities for women have increased, particularly following the Equal Opportunities Act, it has become more difficult to recruit staff.

RECRUITING

The objective of recruiting is to find suitable people to fill vacant posts. It is very important to choose the right person as it can be expensive to:

- recruit – in terms of both time and money;
- make mistakes – if the wrong person is recruited this may lead to conflict and absenteeism;
- provide training to try to improve performance.

Whenever a vacancy arises there is an opportunity to decide if another person is needed in the same role, the type of replacement required or, perhaps, if different expertise is now required. If there is a need to advertise, all recruiting must follow the operational procedure of the organisation as well as employment legislation. A checklist provided by the 'Equal Opportunities Commission 2006' covers the various acts you need to be aware of such as, for example, the Sex Discrimination Act: **www.eoc.org.uk/PDF/recruitmentandselectionchecklist.pdf**. The checklist also contains some guidance for writing job specifications and advertising.

There are two main organisational approaches to recruitment:

- **Job centred** – the essential activities of the job, the expertise and the person characteristics are defined and the advertisement is placed.
- **Placement approach** – staff who should be suitable to join the organisation are hired and training is provided, after which the staff are placed in an appropriate job. For example, NHS management trainees are recruited this way.

Reflection

The placement approach is common in large US health organisations. The personnel department hires suitable staff then phones the managers who have vacancies to tell them that 'we have a warm body'. Individual managers then interview for their own area. This is not a common practice in the UK.

1. What do you need to take into account when recruiting new staff? (See Managing Human Resources and Recruiting.)

Developing a person specification

This should be an essential part of the recruitment process but, while it might appear to be an obvious step, it is often 'skipped'. The most accurate person specification information is supplied by the person who is currently in the role or by their immediate supervisor. To avoid subjectivity it is best to use more than one person's view when drawing up a specification.

The person specification requirements should be divided into those requirements that are essential and those that are desirable. It is important to guard against the idea that there is one ideal candidate for the job. In fact, there is usually a range of people able to fill the role. Employers must ensure that they adhere to employment legislation. Criminal record checks are required when working with vulnerable people and in some jobs, such as nursing, 'spent' criminal records exclude employment (see **www.crb.gov.uk**). You must exclude anything from your specification that could lead to gender, racial and age discrimination. However, a candidate's medical condition should be taken into account when considering them for a job where, for example, a condition like uncontrolled epilepsy might compromise patient/client safety (see **www.opsi.gov.uk/si/si2006/2006 1031.htm#7**).

Reflection

If you want to employ a staff nurse then the essential qualifications would be nurse registration and a record of honesty. If you are recruiting for a specific department then the specialist skills could also be an essential requirement for the job. However, if there were relatively few people available with the required skills, the specific skills may become a desirable characteristic, rather than a requirement, and the nurse would be given training after employment.

1. Review your person specifications. Are they up-to-date with regard to the latest legislation? (See Developing a person specification.)

A role analysis

A role analysis should be written up as a job description and information provided about:

- the specific tasks involved in the role;
- how the tasks should be performed (for managerial jobs there is usually a list of the responsibilities of the role rather than the tasks required);
- the standards of performance, which can then be used to evaluate performance;
- the authority the individual will be allocated.

Advertising

When you are advertising a role you need to consider the following issues.

The local employment market

An employer should know the local market. Are there people available locally with the required skills for the role or do you need to advertise more widely?

Internal or external advertising?

You need to decide where you are going to advertise – internally or externally? In some organisations roles are always advertised internally before they are advertised externally as a matter of course. However, it is important to adhere to equal opportunities legislation and jobs above a certain seniority should always be advertised nationally.

Which is the best place to advertise?

Which papers or journals are best for your purposes – local papers, the national press or specialist journals? National advertising is the most expensive, so it is important to choose the appropriate journal and advertise in the relevant section. For example, if you want a learning disability worker, you will get few replies if the advertisement appears in the mental health section.

Recruiting from overseas

You may need to recruit overseas staff so you will need to be aware of the methods needed to reach your required nationality and you also need to understand the Home Office requirements concerning work permits.

Designing your advertisement

Advertising is an opportunity to sell your organisation and your advertisement should be phrased to entice the right people to apply. It should also be accurate, give a short description of the area of work, what is expected in the job, the essential requirements, the terms and conditions of employment and the deadline for applications. The layout of an advertisement should be done professionally. Some advertisements describe attractive features of the local area, but candidates will be wary when the surrounding countryside is described but not the job itself.

Dealing with prospective candidates

It is important to ensure that prospective candidates are dealt with promptly and efficiently, and that equity is ensured. For many their application will be their first contact with your organisation and you want to give a good impression and stimulate their interest. Also, unfair and unequal treatment of applications can occur inadvertently. For instance, if all job applications have to be online this will exclude those without access to a computer and broadband.

Key Learning Points

Recruitment and selection can be managed by:

- Managing your human resources;
- Being aware of different approaches to recruitment;
- Being aware of discrimination legislation;
- Ensuring you have performed a job analysis;
- Advertising in appropriate ways and knowing the job market.

APPLICATION FORMS

It is worth reviewing your application forms at regular intervals. They can be poorly designed, look boring, be complicated and/or difficult to complete. CVs may not include all the information you need about a candidate so, if you want a completed application form as well as a CV, explicit instructions should be given. This website provides an excellent example of a clear application process: **www.scie.org.uk/recruitment/forms/guidance.doc**. When reviewing your application forms you must check if they adhere to the latest legislation. If you are asking for someone of a specific gender or age to apply you will need to be able to justify this decision.

> ## Reflection
>
> Some of you will have applied to organisations which have been slow to send out an application form or reluctant to reply to your queries. It is rare nowadays for organisations to send a letter telling a candidate they have not been shortlisted. However, I would suggest that a candidate is more likely to apply for another job in your organisation if you do send an acknowledgement of their application.
>
> 1. Do applicants for posts in your organisation know exactly what the post is and what they need to do in order to apply? (See A role analysis, Advertising and Application Forms.)

SHORTLISTING

Time should be taken to create a shortlist that is as objective as possible. Also, if possible, all interviewers should be involved in drawing up the shortlist. In large organisations where the applicants send their completed forms to HR departments, personnel may only forward the forms from those applicants who have the essential requirements for the job. However, transferable skills can be very useful and should be taken into account when shortlisting. When you are shortlisting it can also be helpful to write down a list of the queries that are raised by the information given on the application form, such as queries about gaps in employment.

> ## Reflection
>
> I needed a health care assistant for a day care centre. It was essential that the person in the role had excellent communication skills. One candidate had had no previous experience of health work, but had sold double glazing. She had excellent communication and people skills.
>
> 1. How do you ensure objectivity and consistency when shortlisting? (See Shortlisting and Developing a person specification.)

THE RECRUITMENT PROCESS

Recruitment is a process and it is important not to omit any of the stages (see Figure 1).

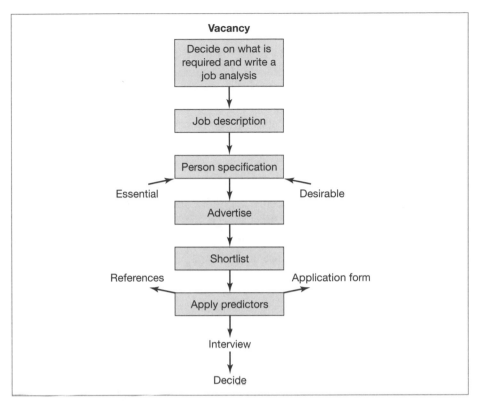

Figure 1 Processes in recruitment and selection

The application form

Gaps in employment in CVs and on application forms should be noted and, if no adequate explanation has been given, questions should be asked at interview. It could be that the candidate has had a period of imprisonment. However, please note that questions should be asked sensitively and candidates should not be excluded inappropriately from employment due to declared past convictions.

References

A key predictor of future performance is, of course, past performance. There are two schools of thought regarding references. Some organisations insist that references are not seen until after interview. This means that all candidates have an equal opportunity to be interviewed. However, it can be argued that few employers are likely to employ someone with two poor references. Other organisations take references into account when shortlisting.

It should be remembered that references are one person's subjective thoughts. For this reason at least two references are sought direct from the referees. 'To whom it may concern' recommendations are sometimes offered by candidates but these should not be taken into consideration as they can easily be forged. It is usual to have a reference from the most recent employer and a reason should be given if the applicant does not want the employer to be contacted. Sometimes the two references do not agree on substantive issues and, if this is the case, then it is usual to ask the candidate at interview for a suitable third referee.

Reflection

If a person applies for a long academic course it is usual to seek an academic reference, often from their training school/college. I once had an appalling academic reference sent for a prospective student from a hospital school of nursing by a chief nurse. The reference had been given ten years previously when the candidate had completed training. It was prefaced with the following words from the chief nurse, who did not know the candidate: 'This is a poor reference. I would suggest if this person is still employed in nursing, that this reference should be disregarded.' We asked for and got a third reference and the student successfully completed the course.

1. Do you have a policy regarding references? When do you refer to them and how many do you ask for? (See References.)

Analysing references

References are often revealing in what they omit, particularly now that employees can ask to see them. Most people writing references want to be honest and fair both to the worker and to the next employer. It is important to give a clear indication of the strengths as well as a fair indication of weaknesses in a reference, as well as offering some suggestions for what could be done to help to develop the person in question. For example, it is important to realise that, just because a person has not shown any leadership qualities while they were employed by you, they may actually have the potential to develop leadership qualities in another setting. This should be highlighted in their reference. With different experience, in a different type of job and with other opportunities, the person concerned may show different qualities. A good example of someone reaching their potential in altered circumstances was Winston Churchill during the Second World War. However, if all that can be said about a person in a reference is that they are neat and tidy, then this is probably indicative of other unmentioned problems.

Reflection

This is an example of a student's reference written at the end of their course: 'Clarry has been a very able mature student who has achieved well in both the clinical area and academically. She tends to be self-deprecating of her attainments, but has worked hard and been determined to succeed. Clarry is a quiet member in a group, but gets on well with other colleagues and patients. Clarry has the ability to do well both in the clinical area and academically. Whilst I think Clarry has the potential to become a leader in a clinical area, she needs to gain further supervised experience.'

1. References should be read alongside your person specification. Does the reference help you to identify development needs? (See Developing a person specification, A role analysis and References.)

Personality clashes will occur between managers and members of staff and personal problems may also affect a person's performance. Sometimes a person can be appointed to a job for which they are unsuitable yet, in another organisation with supportive managers, they may well perform excellently. Some referees 'damn with faint praise' while others try to get rid of an employee by effusively praising them. All of these factors should be considered when reading and writing references.

Issues arising from references

It is usual to ask for information from referees about the number of days off sick and the number of occasions that an employee has been absent over a period of, usually, two years in their present employment. If sickness has occurred in large blocks this could be an indication of an ongoing chronic problem and a medical opinion will probably be needed before the person can be employed. If the periods of sickness have been odd days on numerous occasions, this could also be a sign that the employee has medical problems and, again, it is wise to check. Chronic illnesses should not exclude employment but it is wise to ensure that the person can do the job for which you want to employ them. It could be that a person has a physical complaint that would not be a difficulty if they had a less arduous job or if they were able to work shorter hours. Of course, candidates' privacy should be respected and, if there are any signs of likely difficulties, a referral should be made to a medical practitioner or occupational health, in order that the applicant be properly assessed for their physical capacity to do the job.

Key Learning Points

Recruiting suitable staff depends on:

- A well-designed application form;
- Thoughtful and careful shortlisting;
- Scrutinising references and being aware of potential issues.

INTERVIEWING

The time and effort that goes into interviewing may vary from, for example, 'trial by sherry' where candidates are introduced to colleagues in a social setting, to all-day interviews and/or 10-minute presentations. Some organisations also use psychological and/or IQ (Intelligence Quotient) testing. This can be done on the interview day or prior to interview. For example, it was very popular to use the DC Test for aspiring student nurses who did not have the required GCSEs. The DC Test was the United Kingdom Central Council for Nursing, Midwifery and Health Visiting (UKCC) entry test for nurses. Care needs to be taken when using such tests, particularly when using those that may have a cultural bias; American tests usually have an English version available. Tests have to be consistently reliable and relevant. Also be aware that Personality and Interest Inventories are low predictors of future performance as often the candidates can see what is wanted by the employer.

Information checks

Candidates should be asked to bring their original academic certificates as it is very easy to 'doctor' a photocopy. It is not uncommon for a grade to be changed, a qualification to be claimed, a registration to have expired (or even forged) and CVs to include inflated claims about qualifications and experience. You should ensure that professionals have a current registration, something that may have been overlooked by the person concerned. There was a recent case in the press of a chief executive of an NHS Trust who was fined for claiming a degree that he did not possess.

Interview formats

It is worth checking the information on the application form again before the actual interview so that you can draw inferences about the suitability of an applicant and draw up a list of questions based on the information provided. Most organisations have a set interview format, even to the point of listing the questions to be asked, to ensure that all candidates are treated equally. It can be difficult to adhere strictly to a list of questions, as a candidate is likely to give extra information in a reply. If you then ask the question in the set format, it may well appear that you have not listened to the previous answer. However, it is important to obtain all the required information as well as checking the queries that have been raised by the application form.

Reflection

Information about courses attended can also be exaggerated. I was once on an interview panel, interviewing someone who had attended the same counselling course as I had. It was two days long when I attended, five days long when he did. I also remember stating to a chief nurse that a candidate for a course had forged her grade on her GCSE certificate. The CN was a bit dismissive, as it was an educational certificate. However, as I pointed out to her, she might take a different view if it had been a forgery of a drug register entry.

1. Do you have a list of interview questions and an idea of the answers you are looking for? (See References, Analysing references and Interviewing.)

To be successful, interviewing requires concentration on the part of the interviewer. For this reason it is best not to interview too many candidates in one session. Four to six candidates should be the optimum number to be interviewed at any one time.

Conduct of the interview

Location and seating arrangements

There is a need to achieve a rapport between interviewer and interviewee as an interview should be a pleasant experience and not an inquisition. If the person is unsuccessful you may not want to deter them from applying for another job when a suitable one is available, and you do not want them to give your organisation negative publicity. For this reason many managers interview in an informal setting such as, for example, around a coffee table. Also, it is important to ensure that the seating does not leave the interviewee feeling at a disadvantage, for example if they are in a chair lower than the interviewers or in a chair that is difficult to get in or out of.

The number of interviewers

It is helpful to have at least two interviewers but, preferably, not more than four or the candidate may feel overwhelmed. If there are two or more interviewers you need to decide who is going to cover which aspects of the interview and/or which questions each will ask. You can then take turns, with one interviewer asking their questions, then the other, with an opportunity for either to come back to check information. With two interviewers, one can observe and watch for 'non-verbal' communication and listen for gaps in answers, which can be filled by further questions. It is essential to listen to the interviewee and to ask the question again or rephrase it if you are uncertain about the interviewee's reply. It is also vital to watch for non-verbal communication, especially when trying to estimate if this is really the type of work the candidate wants to do. For this reason many interviewers do not write up the interview until after the candidate has left the room.

Effective questioning

You should avoid closed questions (i.e. questions that can be answered by a 'yes' or a 'no') unless you are asking about a fact that needs clarifying. Never ask 'leading' questions, such as, 'Do you like people'? Few people being interviewed for a caring job are likely to say 'no'.

Multiple questions, for example 'Why do you want to work in this area? Is it because of your previous experience or is it because you want to move into the district?', should also be avoided. The question 'Why do you want to work in this area?' should elicit some response and this can then be followed up with subsequent questions.

There should also be an opportunity to give information to the candidate and an opportunity for candidates to ask any questions that they have. To be fair to all candidates, mothers of small children should not be asked about their child care arrangements. However, the conditions of work can be stated to all candidates, i.e. they are expected to start work at 7 a.m., holidays are to be taken after negotiation with the other staff in the area, etc. If there are 'family friendly' policies, then all ages and both genders should have access to these.

Avoiding bias

When you are interviewing it is very important to be aware of any biases you may have, such as accent, dress, gender, age, race, etc. However, if the interviewee appears in 'street' fashion it is always worth emphasising the expected dress or uniform that they have to wear at work. There can also be a 'halo' effect, i.e. someone whose appearance is good, interviews well and conforms to your prejudices is not necessarily the best candidate for a specific job. Also beware of contrasting your current candidate with the last candidate; this one might appear good because the last one was totally unsuitable.

SELECTION DECISIONS

Decisions should be made as soon as possible after interviewing and the notes should be written up quickly. The reasons why a person has been chosen for the role should be clearly stated, as should the individual reasons why the other candidates have not been selected. If more than one candidate is suitable, but a decision has to be made, it may help to rank the candidates in order of preference. If your top choice turns down your offer, the second choice can then be offered the job.

It is important that the candidates know what has been decided and each one should be contacted by phone or by letter. Feedback to the unsuccessful candidates should also be offered. Some organisations do not do this, but it can be argued that if candidates have taken the time and trouble to travel for the interview they are at least entitled to some feedback. It may also encourage a failed candidate to apply again if another suitable job is advertised.

Key Learning Points

Appointing suitable staff depends on:

- A planned approach to interviewing;
- Careful information checking;
- Well-conducted interviews;
- Clear selection decisions.

Summary of Key Learning Points

Recruitment and selection can be managed by:

- Managing your human resources;
- Being aware of different approaches to recruitment;
- Being aware of discrimination legislation;
- Ensuring you have performed a job analysis;
- Advertising in appropriate ways and knowing the job market.

Recruiting suitable staff depends on:

- A well-designed application form;
- Thoughtful and careful shortlisting;
- Scrutinising references and being aware of potential issues.

Appointing suitable staff depends on:

- A planned approach to interviewing;
- Careful information checking;
- Well-conducted interviews;
- Clear selection decisions.

Case study 1

Mrs Jane Archer owns two 20-bedded care homes. One home is situated in Ambridge, a village 4 miles from the large town of Borchester. There is only one bus a day to the town at 8 a.m. It returns to the village after 5 p.m. in the evening. The sister home is situated in Borchester. Jane has difficulty in recruiting suitable staff for the Ambridge home but rarely has a vacancy in Borchester.

1. What approaches could be used to improve recruitment in Ambridge?
2. The home manager in Ambridge is nearing retirement age. How could finding a replacement be strategically managed?

Case study 2

Mr Bill Forrest is the manager of a large care home in Chelsea by Sea, a retirement area on the south coast. He has difficulty in maintaining a full establishment of staff in the home. While he does receive some applications in reply to advertisements, few of the applicants are suitable at interview. Rarely does a successful candidate take up a post that is offered. On a couple of occasions recently he has seen people to whom he had offered jobs going into the other large home in the next street in health care assistant's uniform.

1. What would you advise Mr Forrest to do to increase his staffing levels?

Activities

1. Reflect on the last time you had a vacancy. Did you just recruit one of the same? Did you use a job-centred or placement approach? What could be the advantages in reassessing your staffing requirements? (See Managing Human Resources and Recruiting.)
2. Try writing a person specification and a job analysis for your own job. Did you have all the essential requirements when you started the job? Has the job changed since you have been in it? (See Developing a person specification and A role analysis.)

3. Have you ever participated in shortlisting? What were the factors you took into account? Did you feel the process you undertook was fair and objective? (See Application Forms, Shortlisting, references, analysing references, Issues arising from references.)

4. Remember your last interview. Was it a pleasant experience? If so, what did you enjoy? If not, what would you had done if you had been the interviewer? (See Interviewing, Information checks, Interview formats, Conduct of the interview.)

5. If you have ever been an interviewer, have you validated the procedure you used? Did your recruit prove to be suitable? Was the procedure worthwhile? If you have not been involved in interviewing, think about how you could validate and evaluate the procedure in your own organisation. (See Interviewing, Information checks, Interview formats, Conduct of the interview, Selection Decisions.)

Chapter 9

Workforce planning and skill mix

INTRODUCTION

The topic of workforce planning and skill mix will enable you to address National Occupational Standards C14 'Manage the performance of team and individuals' and A2 'Manage activities to meet requirements'. In this chapter you will:

- examine how the global picture affects workforce planning in British care environments;
- consider the principles and objectives of workforce planning;
- examine the influences on workforce planning;
- learn how to calculate whole time equivalents (WTE);
- critically examine workforce planning formulas;
- consider the implications and pitfalls of skill mix.

WORKFORCE PLANNING: THE GLOBAL PICTURE

The concept of workforce planning is relatively new in health and social care. Managers are often unconvinced about its use as it seems unpredictable and long-range forecasting can appear unreliable. However, there is a tendency to go from crisis to crisis, especially in nursing and medicine, so a strategic approach to workforce planning should be adopted.

Most professions now form part of a global labour market. This is especially true for nursing and it means that shortages of nurses in Britain can have global implications. Shortages in other countries are also likely to have an impact on Britain because these countries will be looking to recruit staff internationally as well as nationally. For example, a third of US nurses are over the age of 50 (Steinbrook, 2002) and the American Registered Nurse (RN) workforce is expected to be 20 per cent below requirements by 2020 (Buerhaus *et al*, 2000). Evidence from Canada suggests a workforce shortfall of 78,000 nurses by 2011 (Buchan and Seccombe, 2003). It is important for every organisation to try to ensure their recruitment, retention and manpower strategies provide them with sufficient staff. Efforts must also be made to provide satisfactory career structures for qualified nurses so that they do not leave the country or the profession.

PRINCIPLES AND OBJECTIVES OF WORKFORCE PLANNING

People are the most valuable and flexible resource an organisation possesses. Ensuring that your organisation employs the right number of staff with the right skills is fundamental to its success in various ways. For example, the size of the wage bill can be vital when competing for contracts. Also, if you spend time and money finding out what motivates your staff and then providing this motivation, doing so will reduce the need for recruitment, which is far more costly and time-consuming. The objective of workforce planning is therefore to secure human resources on a long-term basis and ensure:

- the recruitment of sufficient and suitable staff;
- that the organisation has the ability to retain staff;
- there is optimal utilisation of staff;
- an improvement in staff performance;
- staff can be disengaged if necessary;
- the quality and quantity of staff can be taken into account;
- human resource policies are integrated in planning so that you avoid possible inconsistencies.

If you don't plan your workforce you risk incurring indirect social costs such as, for example:

- staff becoming frustrated if their promotion hopes are thwarted;
- a failure to adapt and develop skills;
- problems caused by industrial relations issues;
- the need for redundancies.

Some of the inherent problems in workforce planning can be overcome if it is remembered that:

- it does not give a once-and-for-all figure for the number of staff you need;
- the plan needs constant revision;
- the plan is only as good as the information that is used to create it.

The psychological/social contract

There used to be an unspoken psychological/social contract that employees made with an organisation. In return for commitment to the firm and performing well in their job they expected promotion and an assured future. The contract was reciprocally renewed at intervals throughout an employee's career. Flatter structures, with less hierarchy, are changing this contract as there are fewer opportunities for promotion. Organisations now require staff to accept that redundancy and early retirement are more likely than career advancement, with middle managers being the most affected. With organisational changes, particularly in areas where staff have been made redundant, the psychological/social contract with an employer may have changed. There is no longer a job for life and individuals are now expected to plan their own careers. Organisations should also prepare staff flexibly for the jobs that are likely to be developed. It is said that, during their career, every employee in the health service will work in three jobs that were not in existence when they started work.

In all workforce planning exercises there is a need to incorporate and analyse many factors.

THE PROCESS OF WORKFORCE PLANNING

The process of workforce planning is inextricably linked to the corporate aims of an organisation. Planning must also be examined in the context of a specific social, political and economic environment. There is a tendency to make the process appear scientific but it is still based on guesswork as many factors are unknown. For example, future needs will be:

- influenced by factors like changes in technology;
- affected by changes in employment law, such as working hours directives.

Unless planning is undertaken consistently, management may not notice long-term trends until there is a crisis, which could then result in:

- an inadequate supply of key workers;
- low morale;
- high turnover;
- career blockages.

When planning, it is best to start with the information that you already have. For example, you can estimate when staff are likely to retire by examining their dates of birth, particularly in known shortage areas. Those eligible for early retirement at 55 may be encouraged to stay on, either on a full-time or part-time basis. Newly qualified staff are also likely to move on after they have gained experience. If new services are to be provided or a new building is constructed, the staffing requirements can be estimated. Previous staffing trends can be extrapolated, with the proviso that they may not hold true again.

Reflection

I was working as a regional educational contractor and suggested to an acute hospital Trust that perhaps they could examine the likely recruitment needs in some of their shortage areas. They looked at the dates of birth of their staff in their special care baby unit (SCBU) and found that most of the staff were due to retire within the next two years. As it takes at least six months to acquire the specialised skills required, they needed either to train members of their existing staff as replacements, recruit staff with the necessary skills, or recruit staff that they could train.

In another Trust, I was asked if there were any courses available for adolescent mental health staff and had to admit there were none in the region. It usually takes about a year to set up a new course, to get it written, validated and recruit a tutor, and then staff have to undertake the course. I asked why there was a sudden need for staff and was told that a new unit was nearing completion and would be ready for use in six weeks' time. No staff were available within the Trust with the necessary qualifications. It had taken 18 months to build the unit and no one during that period had thought about how they were going staff it.

1. Does your organisation undertake any workforce planning? If not, why not? If it does, what does the planning consist of? Does it work? (See Principles and Objectives of Workforce Planning and The Process of Workforce Planning.)

Information available for workforce planning

A wide range of information is available to support the process of workforce planning.

The number of health and social care workers in training

National and local figures for the number of students and practitioners in training are available. Check with the Nursing and Midwives Council for nurses in training and Skills for Care and CSCI for the numbers of care workers in training.

Age

If it is usual in your organisation to recruit females at 18 years old, then it is important to examine both national and local demographic trends to see how the number of 18-year-old females changes over time.

Gender

Again, the local and national trends for gender numbers can be examined.

Occupation

In some areas there may be few people living locally who are available for recruitment with the qualifications you require. In the short term this may mean that you have to recruit nationally. In the long term it would be sensible to recruit untrained staff or, if at all possible, help to set up courses to enable people to obtain qualifications locally. For information on age, gender and occupation, check **www.statistics.gov.uk**.

Qualifications

Check the qualifications of your current staff members. It may be that some people have specialist qualification certificates but are currently working in other areas.

Sickness levels

Sickness levels can be calculated from the information you have available in your organisation.

Staff turnover

Staff turnover can also be calculated for your department and organisation. The average turnover of staff and average length of time that a member of staff stays in the organisation can be calculated. The longer staff stay, the greater the reduction in costs for recruitment. However, there can be disadvantages in that staff can become static and reluctant to embrace new ideas.

Areas that are difficult to recruit for

Areas that are difficult to recruit for include the care of the elderly, psychiatric care and learning disabilities. Providing incentives such as educational opportunities could help recruitment in these areas.

Demand for your organisation's goods and services

Information about the likely demand for your organisation's goods and services is often known in advance, so recruitment or forward training can be planned.

Skills shortages

There can be national and/or local skills shortages in certain areas, which will mean that training is needed for all recruits in these areas.

Technology changes

Some changes in technology may be known about and can be planned for. Other changes may be forecast so you will need to stay in touch with these and try to anticipate the impact they may have on your organisation.

Time

It takes time to train a professional. Nurses and allied health professionals will, on average, spend three years on a course. The process of commissioning student places takes a year, which means that at least four years must be allowed before the professional is ready to start work.

Geographical area

Information is available on issues like:

- other competition for workforce in your local area, such as shopping centres;
- national and regional trends in population;
- the per cent of registered nurses over the age of 40 (NMC figures);
- the economic situation; for example, if there is a downturn in the local economy then more males may be attracted to nursing and care work;
- the cost of local housing may make it difficult to recruit locally.

Political changes

Be aware of political changes that may affect workforce planning such as:

- government schemes/policies;
- population movements – migration internally and externally;
- policies on topics like redundancy payments, etc.

Not much can be done to influence either the geographic or the political situation locally or nationally, but it should be considered and when plans are made, the obvious problems that are likely to occur should be taken into account.

Reflection

I was once involved with recruiting for a school of nursing. At the time, we were the only school in the county that managed to ensure that we had our full complement of students. One of the hospitals that we served was in a very depressed area and the local schooling provision left a lot to be desired. This meant that it was difficult to recruit local people into training as they did not have the required academic qualifications. However, it was very easy to recruit mature health care assistants (HCAs) as there was little other work available that was not seasonal. We had an understanding with and encouragement from the Director of Nursing to recruit suitable HCAs into training as, on completion of their training, many of the locals then remained in the area. To assist in recruitment we asked the local further education college to run a course in literacy, numeracy and communication skills, paid for by each HCA, and at the end of the course they undertook the DC test (an IQ test) and were then taken into training. Local research showed that these students had a higher completion rate than conventional students and an average academic achievement. This was just one of the strategies we used to keep our school full.

1. Are you aware of the local conditions regarding issues: for example, demographics and education opportunities? How would you find this information? (See Information available for workforce planning.)

Key Learning Points

Planning the workforce requires:

• An understanding of the global market;
• An awareness of the principles and objectives of workforce planning;
• An understanding of the processes of workforce planning;
• An awareness of the factors affecting workforce planning.

ANALYSING YOUR WORKFORCE

Establishments (Hurst K. 2002)

Establishments of wards, departments and care homes have been historically set at a basis of a bed occupancy of 85 per cent. However, establishments did not necessarily take into account client dependency or the skills of the staff and, once set, it was often the case that they were not altered regularly to take account of any changes. If wards were transferred to new buildings (for example, from a nightingale-type ward to one with cubicles or single rooms) the need for extra staff was not always reviewed. Throughout the 1970s and 1980s there were increasing problems with recruitment, which became even more urgent in the 1990s when there was a dramatic drop in the population of the traditional source of nurse recruits – 18-year-old females. For these reasons, workforce planning became more necessary and it is now clear that establishments should be analysed on a regular basis.

You can analyse the establishment as follows. The 'numbers in post' are the numbers of staff actually employed in the area. Numbers of staff in post are normally smaller than establishments and a comparison of the two gives the vacancy rate, which can be expressed in percentage terms.

$$100 - \frac{(\text{number in post (NIP)})}{\text{Establishment (E)}} \times 100 = \text{vacancy rate}$$

e.g. $100 - \frac{\text{NIP} 20}{\text{E } 25} \times 100 = 20\%$

Working out Whole Time Equivalents (WTEs)

Staffing is usually measured in WTEs. This enables like to be compared with like, particularly when, as in nursing or the care sector, many staff are part time. A full-time staff member, i.e. one who works 37.5 hours a week, is counted as 1.0. A staff member who works 20 hours is 0.53 WTE. To calculate the WTE:

$$\text{WTE} = 20 \div 37.5 = 0.53 \text{ WTE}$$

If a full-time staff member works 35 hours then this = 1.0, so a staff member who works 20 hours = $20 \div 35 = 0.57$ WTE.

If you do not use WTEs when measuring your staffing, try converting your present staffing using the equation.

WORKFORCE PLANNING SCHEMES

There are five nursing workforce planning schemes:

1. The professional judgement approach.
2. Nurses Per Occupied Bed (NPOB).
3. The acuity/quality method.
4. The timed task/activity report.
5. Regression-based systems.

Look at the following definitions. One or a combination of these schemes probably reflects your approach to workforce planning in the social care sector.

Professional judgement

Telford's (1979) early work uses expert professional judgement to decide on the most appropriate size and mix of a ward nursing team. This method has stood the test of time. To calculate the number of working hours and WTEs needed:

Early shift 0700 to 1430 = 7.5 hours x 3 nurses x 7 days = 157.5 hours

Late shift 1400 to 2130 = 7.5 hours x 3 nurses x 7 days = 157.5 hours

Night shift 2100 to 0715 = 10 hours x 2 nurses x 7 days = 140 hours

Total = 455 hours

Time out for sickness, holidays, etc. = 22% = 455 x 1.22

= 555.1 ÷ 37.5

= 14.8 WTEs

This formula can be varied. For example, a five-day ward would only need 18 per cent time out and for day wards you would only need to cover one shift. Similar adjustments can be made if you are running a day centre or a 24-hour residential care service. The formula can be used to calculate the staff numbers you should have from what you have got, either in available nurses or funded.

Strengths

- A quick and inexpensive scheme.
- It can be applied to any speciality and is easy to update.
- It is often used to check other methods.
- Little adjustment is needed for different care groups.
- New methods of working can be easily accommodated.

Weaknesses

- It is difficult to explain the relationship between quality and staffing levels.
- It is less flexible when client numbers and dependencies change.
- It can be subjective and needs an experienced professional.
- With long shifts calculations can be complex.
- As professional judgement is involved in the decision on staff numbers, funding constraints may influence this judgement.

Nurses Per Occupied Bed (NPOB)

This is a popular method and some of the Royal Colleges have used this to work out the numbers for their specialities. For example, per bed = care of the elderly = 1.21 WTE. In this method holidays come out of establishment. This formula can and, many would argue, should be applied to the nursing home and residential care sector.

Strengths

- Data is easy to benchmark.
- It can be verified by using professional judgement.
- If the bed complement changes it is easy to modify the establishment.
- It is simple to work out workforce planning.
- Formulas vary with specialities.

Weaknesses

- The method assumes that historically staffing has been rationally determined.
- There is little relationship to occupancy.
- There is no guarantee that average staffing produces quality outcomes.
- It is insensitive to client dependency.
- It is costly to update.
- Geographically different wards/care homes require different staffing ratios.

The acuity/quality method

The dependency of clients is taken into account in this method and it can be useful where client numbers fluctuate and there is a mix of clients. A minimum number should be stipulated below which staff numbers should not fall. The calculation is based on a dependency grading:

1 = almost independent
2 = partially independent
3 = partially dependent
4 = totally dependent

Therefore, a Grade 1 client (almost independent) = 46 minutes of nursing time per day. A Grade 4 client (totally dependent) = 336 minutes = 5.6 hours nursing time per day. The calculation also takes into account that, as only 42 per cent of nurses' time is spent in direct care, indirect care needs to be added in thus:

+10% meal and drink breaks;

+22% sick or annual leave.

Seniority, qualifications and experience of staff must also be taken into account.

Strengths

- You can use local data and the method can be used in short-stay situations.
- You can change variables easily.
- You can suit the numbers of clients to the numbers of nurses.
- Benchmarking and performance indicators are easy to calculate.

Weaknesses

- This method can be subjective.
- It is based on a previous shift's dependency gradings.
- It fails to measure psychological care.
- It is difficult to calculate for small wards.
- Additional client information is needed.

The timed task/activity method

In this method the dependency of clients is measured and the categories calculated, for example, Category 1 = self caring and Category 4 = high input (ITU). Significant events such as admission and discharge should also be taken into account and there is a need to identify appropriate grade mixes. There is no set formula for this method as timing is worked out related to planned care, for example, hygiene needs 20 minutes and observations 60 minutes.

Strengths

- This is a good method for calculating staff needs for wards with elective admissions.
- It uses statistical methods – predictions of nursing requirements for future shifts are based on previous shifts.
- It is easily computerised.

Weaknesses

- It is difficult to be objective when measuring dependency because client needs change from one shift to the next.
- This scheme is expensive to set up, it must be reviewed regularly and care plans must be up to date.
- There is a tendency to overestimate as nurses do not do one task at a time.

Regression analysis

This method predicts the number of nurses required for a given level of activity and bed occupancy. Once the base data is acquired it is then straightforward to use a method similar to NPOB, but the services of a statistician may be needed to set up a programme (Hurst K. 2002).

Some final thoughts on planning schemes

- No system provides reliable information and it is possible that none of the methods are valid in that they are not measuring what they purport to measure.
- The objectivity of those operating the schemes can be questionable.
- There is no theoretical basis for the variables that are selected.
- Estimating the timing of activities is only possible using historical data and methods of giving care change.
- Activities are added linearly – neither multitasking nor the skills of nurses are taken into account.
- Care plans are often inaccurate.
- Prioritising takes place.
- There is a tendency to work harder and faster until the limit is reached.
- Clients are more homogeneous now – most are very sick. In the past there would have been more of a mix of independent and dependent clients, so it should be easier to estimate data these days.
- In fact, professional judgement is as accurate as any of the other methods used (RCN, 2001).

There are pressures on staffing and the main one is increasing costs. Twenty-four-hour care over seven days a week is labour intensive, so the budget for staffing is usually about 70–75 per cent of total costs. Any wage increases, or increases in staffing numbers, represent large sums of money, so when there are financial pressures to cut costs the staffing budget is the first to be targeted. The tendency is to think that if a total of 105.5 WTE is employed, no one will miss the 0.5. In reality, the area that has 20 fewer hours of care does miss the carer. It should be remembered that, prior to the introduction of Project 2000 nurse training, 30 per cent of all nursing was provided by students. Getting the figures wrong can also be an expensive business. Trusts spent £2.5m, on average, for bank and agency staff in 1999/2000.

Key Learning Points

Estimating the number of workers you require means:

- Understanding WTEs and the factors involved in their calculation;
- A critical awareness of different workforce planning schemes and their strengths and weaknesses.

SKILL MIX

There is a tendency to think of skill mix as a method of diluting the skills of the staff. While in some areas trained staff members have been replaced by untrained staff, a review of skill mix should really be considered as an opportunity to ensure that each area employs the necessary staff with the required qualifications and experience for the work. It may be necessary to revise the skill level upwards, particularly in areas where the type of clients in care have more acute conditions or require more care. There is also a need to distinguish Grade/Band mix from skill mix. For example, in nursing a person may have a G grade (Band 7: ward manager level) but may not have the specific skills (a specialist qualification) required for a specific area. Two measures should be examined:

1. **Optimum skill mix** – this can be estimated, but there is also a need to ascertain the quality required. There has to be an agreement on acceptable and achievable levels of care. It is essential to evaluate the care being given (Richardson, 1999).
2. **Economic skill mix** – good quality has economic implications so, practically, it is important to set the standards. While it would be ideal for every client to have a carer, this is rarely feasible. The costs of care increase with the cost of living.

There has to be an agreement on the achievable levels of care and their acceptability, remembering that quality has costs.

There is also a need to distinguish between the levels of skills. It is common to call certain tasks basic and then allocate them to assistants. It should be remembered that, while some tasks can be safely allocated if supervision is provided, the quality of care improves if qualified staff deliver care (Carr-Hill *et al*, 1992). However, in Britain few organisations use any of the staffing formulas on a regular basis, leading Audit Scotland to comment:

With few exceptions, there is little guidance on the appropriate level of nurse staffing, and levels have historically been determined on the basis of experience and professional judgement.

(Audit Scotland, 2002, p. 15)

This is despite the findings of Carr-Hill *et al.* (1992), who concluded:

- Grade mix had an effect on the quality of care – better quality of care is given by higher-grade nurses.
- Variation in standards were reduced when higher-grade staff worked with lower-grade staff.
- Better outcomes were associated with a higher proportion of registered staff.
- There is a need to develop effective methods of organising nursing care.
- Unplanned uncoordinated care can be wasteful.
- Where overall staffing and the proportion of qualified nurses is low in relation to workload only the basic physical needs of clients can be met.

Research from the United States has shown that clients have shorter stays, fewer complications and fewer infections when there is a higher ratio of registered staff (Currie *et al*, 2005). The state of California, in an endeavour to prevent medical errors, has attempted to impose mandated nurse staffing ratios (Bolton *et al*, 2001; ICN, 2002) and there are also moves to identify research priorities in the quality of care and staffing levels in nursing homes (Kovner *et al*, 2000). Some aspects of care do have suggested ratios but there appears to have been little research done into ratios of care staff to residents in care homes.

Key Learning Points

Working out optimum skill mix requires:

- A knowledge of the needs of your clients;
- An understanding of skill levels and the importance of supervision.

Summary of Key Learning Points

Planning the workforce requires:

- An understanding of the global market;
- An awareness of the principles and objectives of workforce planning;
- An understanding of the processes of workforce planning;
- An awareness of the factors affecting workforce planning.

Estimating the number of workers you require means:

- Understanding WTEs and the factors involved in their calculation;
- A critical awareness of different workforce planning schemes and their strengths and weaknesses.

Working out optimum skill mix requires:

- A knowledge of the needs of clients;
- An understanding of skill levels and the importance of supervision.

Case study 1

Mrs Rose Thornton is a manager of a nursing home in the south-east of England. The owners of the home would like to expand their business and want to build a home in an adjacent commuting town. The whole area has been earmarked as a regeneration area and there are plans to build 30,000 new homes. Rose has been asked by the owners to draw up a two-year workforce plan for both the new home and her present home.

1. What factors should she take into account?

Case study 2

Jane Crow is working in a 20-bed residential home, which has recently become a nursing home. While a few more care assistants were taken on as staff when the home changed its designation, the establishment of the home was not changed and there have subsequently been problems with care.

1. What method/s could be used to calculate the skill mix of staff needed to ensure sufficient expertise is available at any time?

Activities

1. Reflect on your psychological/social contract with your employer. What do you expect from them? Is it a job for life or is it an opportunity to enhance your skills either in your present job, through promotion or a sideways move? Have your expectations changed over the last couple of years? If so, why? (See The psychological/social contract.)

2. What is your establishment? What is your vacancy factor? Is this higher than normal? At what grades/levels do you have vacancies? (See Establishments.)
3. What method do you use, or has your organisation used, to calculate staffing requirements? (See Workforce Planning Schemes.)
4. Examine your care environment. What is the skill mix? Is it appropriate for the numbers and types of clients? If not, what would be appropriate? (See Skill Mix.)

Chapter 10

Financial management

INTRODUCTION

The topic of financial management will enable you to address National Occupational Standard B3 'Manage the use of financial resources'. In this chapter you will:

- consider the principles of budgeting;
- enhance your awareness of financial codes and practices;
- improve your budgeting skills;
- understand the principles of writing a business plan;
- understand the basics of contracting.

DEFINITIONS AND PRINCIPLES OF BUDGETING

A budget is an annual formalised plan that compares income (revenue) with expenses (costs). It is a quantitative statement of a plan to achieve given objectives. Many in the caring professions say that they do not understand budgets, but if you can understand your pay slip there should be no difficulty in understanding a budget report. Budgets:

- provide a plan for the future;
- increase communication – requirements are evident from the figures;
- can provide motivation if the challenge is achievable, but can demotivate if the budget is too difficult to achieve;
- can show performance;
- can be used to control costs.

Reflection

I inherited a budget in the third month of a financial year. It was already £18,000 overspent. I realised that the money allocated for staff pay was £62,000 less than staff would earn over the year. I could only see three alternatives: a) be overdrawn, b) sack staff or c) try to make up the deficit. As I only had money in the budget for staff pay, drugs and medical surgical supplies, it would be impossible to use the third option. I went to see the Director of Finance and explained. I was told it was my problem and I had to come in within budget. A new Director of Finance was then appointed. I went to see him and explained my problem. His solution was for me to come in £50,000 overdrawn so I had to find £12,000. This was achievable and was therefore a good motivator.

1. Are you responsible for a budget? If not, ask to see a copy of the budget of your unit or care home and use this as background for this chapter. If you have a budget, do you find that it motivates or demotivates you? Explain why this is.

The principles of budgeting

There are four main principles in budgeting:

- Money cannot be spent twice.
- Some money should be put aside for emergencies.
- Adhere to the organisation's financial code.
- Value for money – use the budget to provide the best care for the money available.

If these principles are adhered to, providing the emergencies are not excessive, the bottom line of the budget should be in the black rather than in the red. Increasing your ability to manage a budget sheet does not mean that you will get more money (Iles, 1997), but it should enable you to use the money you have been allocated wisely, to achieve your objectives and improve your services.

Money cannot be spent twice

It should be self-evident that money cannot be spent twice. In my experience, I find that where budgeting is concerned even quite senior staff appear to think that they can spend the same money on two different things. You do not have a credit card issued with a budget; you cannot get credit so you must keep within the amount agreed.

Reflection

Reflect on your budget at home. If you spend all your money on treats or clothes, you cannot spend it on food. In a care environment if all the money is spent on medical and surgical supplies, you may have to economise on staff numbers.

Money for emergencies

Keeping an amount of money back for emergencies is vital. For example, if you have equipment such as hoists, they may need repair/replacement during a year. If possible, some money needs to be retained to ensure all equipment can be kept in working order throughout the year. If, at the end of the year, there is a surplus, it can be used to buy new equipment.

Reflection

When working in a school of nursing I was in charge of allocating the audio-visual budget. It was allocated to two areas: the acute team of tutors and the mental health team of tutors. The money was allocated pro rata for the number of students for which each team was responsible. I would notify the mental health team of the amount of their allocation and ask them for their requests. Each year I would get requests totalling more than the allocation. I would send them back, restating the amount of money that was available. This would happen several times before I would get requests within the budget. I would also point out that money needed to be set aside for any repairs as there was no separate pot of money for this. Despite this, each year the mental health team would ask for money for repairs during the year and eventually repair their equipment when the next year's allocation was distributed. For much of the year they could not use their equipment. The acute nursing team's budget was managed, equipment repaired and, at the end of the year, any surplus we had was spent on new equipment.

1. Does your manager attempt to keep some money aside in the budget for repairs/emergencies? If not, what happens when equipment needs repair? (See The principles of budgeting.)

Financial codes and practices

Each organisation should have written financial principles and practices. In the public domain it should be remembered that all money has to be accounted for and all practices should be transparent. While the regulations concerning public liability can lead to complaints of 'excessive red tape', it is important to ensure that you adhere to the regulations. Be aware that financial impropriety can be a 'dismissing offence', and it is vital to ensure that everything you sign for is correct to your knowledge. This is important when, for example, dealing with staff expense claims. It is easy to prove excessive expenditure on claims as the figures speak for themselves.

Reflection

I discovered, on taking a service manager's job, that I was expected to countersign staff time sheets for the entire directorate's nursing staff. As I did not work directly with the staff and was not present at weekends I did not know if the time sheets were correct. While few staff would knowingly put in false claims, it was easy to make a mistake and it would be difficult for me to detect. I asked the ward managers to countersign the sheets as they worked directly with the staff and should have accurate records at ward level.

1. Do you check everything (stores, drugs, time sheets, etc.) for which you sign? If not, why not? (See The principles of budgeting and Financial codes and practices.)

Value for money

It is important to have a clear idea of what value for money is in your area. Is it quality of care? Is it throughput? (See the Information and Quality chapter, page 169.) What is expected in terms of value for money should be clarified and made evident to all members of staff working in the area. It should also be remembered that quality costs money. Having more staff on duty costs money but having fewer staff on duty, while apparently costing less, can lead to poor care, which can actually cost more for each patient's stay.

Key Learning Points

The important issues regarding the management of your budget include:

- Being aware of the principles of budgeting – for example, money cannot be spent twice;
- Understanding and applying financial codes and practices relevant to the public domain;
- Having a clear view of what 'value for money' is in relation to your care environment.

BUDGETING SKILLS

When you are given a budget it is essential to take time to understand a) how all the expenditure that appears on your budget sheets will be incurred and b) how all the income is accrued. Accounting information is used both inside and outside an organisation. Inside an organisation it is management accounting used for decision making. Outside an organisation financial accounting is required for regulatory purposes (Iles, 1997). Financial accounting is written by accountants for accountants on an annual basis and it is expected that, unless non-accountants have had training, they will require help to understand the accounts. Management accounting is for internal use and it can be provided in any format that is useful to the organisation. It is an ongoing performance report, presenting the present and future financial state of the separate parts of an organisation, such as ward or department budget reports. The budget report should state actual accomplishments and planned performance, with any discrepancies clearly marked (Iles, 1997). Improving your budgeting skills should enable you to:

- analyse your costs;
- understand how management decisions will affect your budget position;
- monitor your performance.

Budgeting skills are essential for managers as finance is a resource which has to be managed in conjunction with your other resources.

Costs

Costs during the year include the following items.

Direct costs

Wages and the equipment used in your area. These costs are within your control.

Indirect costs

These are costs that are incurred over several areas of the organisation, for example, rubbish collection. You cannot control the indirect costs for other parts of the business but you can control your department's contribution to them. The total indirect costs for the organisation can be divided into the various parts of the organisation that are incurring them. This gives more control over indirect costs to individual managers.

Overheads

Overheads are organisational costs that include items like the capital costs of, for example, running the building. You cannot control the overheads outside those of your own area of the organisation.

Variable costs

Variable costs change (vary) in direct relation to the amount of activity (see Figure 1). If you increase your activity, your costs increase. For example, if the number of service users increases then you will need more medical supplies.

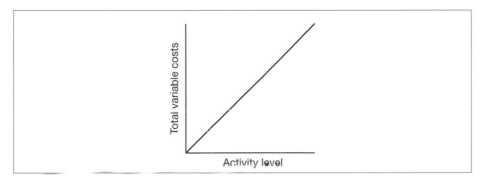

Figure 1 Variable costs (Iles, 1997, p. 70)

Fixed costs

Fixed costs remain the same regardless of the amount of activity (see Figure 2). They are fixed over time (usually one year) but can be recurrent. For example, the salary of a nurse is fixed regardless of the amount of activity that is undertaken. If, however, you have fewer patients, then the cost per patient rises, as the same costs have to be apportioned to a smaller number of patients. No cost is completely fixed as, for example, staff numbers can be increased or staff can be dismissed.

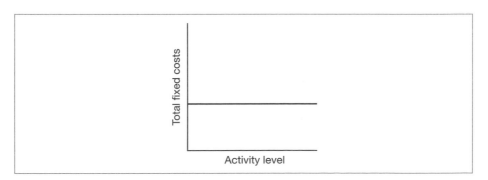

Figure 2 Fixed costs (Iles, 1997, p. 70)

Average costs

The average cost is the mean cost of individual expenditure on, for example, food. The average cost applies to both fixed and variable costs, which can be divided by, for example, the number of patients.

Marginal costs

Marginal costs are the additional costs of a unit after fixed costs have been accounted for. For example, blood tests will cost a certain amount but, once the capital costs, equipment and staff costs have been covered then the cost of any future tests will be marginal.

Relevant costs

If money has already been committed to a project or a piece of equipment then its cost is irrelevant as that money has been put aside.

Opportunity costs

Opportunity costs are hypothetical but relevant in that the value benefit has been forgone. Therefore, by taking the opportunity to use money for one activity, such as occupational therapy rather than another activity such as employing extra nurses, the opportunity cost is that you cannot have more nurses, i.e. you cannot have both nurses and occupational therapists. You may have to work out the opportunity costs in situations where there are limited resources.

Capital investment

Capital is the money spent on major equipment and buildings; things which the organisation owns and where the benefits of ownership last longer than a year and/or the initial cost is over a prescribed limit.

Variance

Variance is the difference between the amount allocated and the amount spent. If you have £12,000 allocated for catering but only spend £9,500, the difference of £2,500 is a variance. If this is due to being able to find a cheaper reliable supplier, then it could be a saving. If it is due to underfeeding patients this could lead to prosecution. Budgets should be flexible and it should be feasible to change money from one heading to another throughout the financial year. In reality it can be difficult and you may need to wait until the budget is renegotiated (normally annually) to reallocate monies (Iles, 1997).

Reflection

The problems of variance with expenditure can show up due to changes in treatment. For example, if a new antibiotic is introduced that treats MRSA, it may be very expensive to provide and the drug budget will then be overspent. However, the fact that patients can be discharged quicker and are less likely to infect others will be a significant advantage. Unfortunately, only the expense of the drug will show up on the ward/department budget report and not the advantages.

1. Examine recent budgets in your care environment. What causes the largest variance in costs? Is there anything that could be done to reduce the variance? (See Costs.)

CONTROLLING EXPENDITURE

It is important to monitor expenditure on your budget report or you may have sleepless nights. Managing a budget is part of the manager's role. It is therefore imperative that you gain sufficient skills to ensure that you do control expenditure, or you may have to make unpalatable choices such as making staff redundant. It is also essential to have the skills to ensure that only your department's costs occur on your budget report. Finance departments have been known to misallocate budgets and this will increase your costs unnecessarily.

Reflection

When ordering supplies it is essential to use the correct cost code for your area. I was once told about two medical wards in a Trust. Despite attempting to drastically cut expenditure one ward was always in financial trouble for overspending on supplies. The other was always being praised for being financially prudent. It took some time for all concerned to realise that the underspending ward was using the wrong cost code. Much of its expenditure was being allocated to the other ward.

If you are responsible for a budget, you should also be involved in setting it. You should know your area and the difficulties you have had with the previous year's budget, as well as the likely changes in care/treatments/equipment that may occur in the near future. In some organisations it can be difficult for a departmental manager to understand the pressures on an organisation, so a 'top down' approach to budgeting may be used. Allocation of funds within an organisation can mean that some departments may gain while others lose and this can affect operational activity if it is not done carefully.

> ## Reflection
>
> Organisations often have historical budget allocations that have been influenced by the 'political pull' of the medical staff. One hospital in a Trust had five consultants and increased staffing levels on care of the elderly wards. The other hospital had two consultants and poor staffing levels. The proportion and numbers of elderly in the local population was in fact higher in the area which had two consultants. It was difficult to reallocate resources in the short term.
>
> 1. Examine your budget. Is the money evenly spread? If one area has more resources than another, is this justified? (See Controlling Expenditure.)

Key Learning Points

Budgeting skills include:

- Understanding how to manage your expenditure;
- Understanding differences in costs (for example, direct and indirect costs) and how to control your costs by controlling expenditure.

APPROACHES TO BUDGETING

There are two main approaches to budgeting:

1. **Incremental budgeting** – costs are increased on the previous year in line with inflation, price and wages rises and the effect of any planned projects, as well as any expected savings.
2. **Zero-based budgeting** – a budget is constructed from first principles. All activity is examined, core activity determined and decisions made as to what, if any, of the other activity previously carried out will continue. Costs are updated and allowances made for any planned projects. Zero-based budgeting is financially better practice, but is time consuming and it is difficult for inexperienced managers to know all the aspects involved.

Budget reports

There is a specific financial vocabulary used in most budget reports, though the layout of a budget report will often differ depending on the organisation.

Cost centre

A cost centre is a unique number or name that identifies the site, department, ward, etc. and this will normally appear at the top of the report.

Expense head

The expense head identifies type of expenditure. For example, wages, drugs, etc.

Period

The period is the financial period covered by the report. This is not always a calendar year. In the NHS the financial year is April to March of the following year, so April is period 1 and November is period 08. In higher education the financial year may run from September to the following August.

Narrative expressed with account codes

The account code describes the expenditure. Account codes are linked to individual lines in the budget. An account code is the combination of an expense head and cost centre, for example, the pharmacy on a medical ward.

Manpower Equivalent or Whole Time Equivalent (MPE or WTE)

The MPE or WTE staff in post (see Figure 3). To calculate a WTE, divide the actual hours by the standard hours for a full time post $16/37.5 = 0.43$ (see also Chapter 9, page 131). Note that hours paid are not necessarily the same as hours worked because of enhancements. By using WTEs, it is easier to compare like with like in staffing numbers.

Budget this month

Usually the annual budget is divided by the number of periods in a year so that, for example, £22,789 ÷ 12 = £1,900 per month, as this is the pattern in which most of the expenditure is incurred. Where expenditure is not incurred in this way it may be more appropriate to change the pattern. For example, the budget for bills received quarterly should be divided by 4 so that £22,789 ÷ 4 = £5,700. This will prevent the creation of misleading variances. As it is not common for expenditure patterns to be varied like this so managers should be aware of the reasons for variances.

Expenditure this month

The expenditure shown will include the expenditure that has been incurred for the period but not necessarily paid, for example, bills.

Annual budget

The total budget available to provide the service for the year.

Hours/ Week	37 hrs/wk WTE	37.5 hrs/wk WTE	38 hrs/wk WTE	39 hrs/wk WTE	Hours/ Week	37 hrs/wk WTE	37.5 hrs/wk WTE	38 hrs/wk WTE	39 hrs/wk WTE
10.0	0.27	0.27	0.26	0.26	25.0	0.68	0.67	0.66	0.64
10.5	0.28	0.28	0.28	0.27	25.5	0.69	0.68	0.67	0.65
11.0	0.30	0.29	0.29	0.28	26.0	0.70	0.69	0.68	0.67
11.5	0.31	0.31	0.30	0.29	26.5	0.72	0.71	0.70	0.68
12.0	0.32	0.32	0.32	0.31	27.0	0.73	0.72	0.71	0.69
12.5	0.34	0.33	0.33	0.32	27.5	0.74	0.73	0.72	0.71
13.0	0.35	0.35	0.34	0.33	28.0	0.76	0.75	0.74	0.72
13.5	0.36	0.36	0.36	0.35	28.5	0.77	0.76	0.75	0.73
14.0	0.38	0.37	0.37	0.36	29.0	0.78	0.77	0.76	0.74
14.5	0.39	0.39	0.38	0.37	29.5	0.80	0.79	0.78	0.76
15.0	0.41	0.40	0.39	0.38	30.0	0.81	0.80	0.79	0.77
15.5	0.42	0.41	0.41	0.40	30.5	0.82	0.81	0.80	0.78
16.0	0.43	0.43	0.42	0.41	31.0	0.84	0.83	0.82	0.79
16.5	0.45	0.44	0.43	0.42	31.5	0.85	0.84	0.83	0.81
17.0	0.46	0.46	0.45	0.44	32.0	0.86	0.85	0.84	0.82
17.5	0.47	0.47	0.46	0.45	32.5	0.88	0.87	0.86	0.83
18.0	0.49	0.48	0.47	0.46	33.0	0.89	0.88	0.87	0.85
18.5	0.50	0.49	0.49	0.47	33.5	0.91	0.89	0.88	0.86
19.0	0.51	0.51	0.50	0.49	34.0	0.92	0.91	0.89	0.87
19.5	0.53	0.52	0.51	0.50	34.5	0.93	0.92	0.91	0.88
20.0	0.54	0.53	0.53	0.51	35.0	0.95	0.93	0.92	0.90
20.5	0.55	0.55	0.54	0.53	35.5	0.96	0.95	0.93	0.91
21.0	0.57	0.56	0.55	0.54	36.0	0.97	0.96	0.95	0.92
21.5	0.58	0.57	0.57	0.55	36.5	0.99	0.97	0.95	0.94
22.0	0.59	0.59	0.58	0.55	37.0	1.00	0.99	0.97	0.95
22.5	0.61	0.60	0.59	0.58	37.5	–	1.00	0.99	0.96
23.0	0.62	0.61	0.61	0.59	38.0	–	–	1.00	0.97
23.5	0.64	0.63	0.62	0.60	38.5	–	–	–	0.99
24.0	0.65	0.64	0.63	0.62	39.0	–	–	–	1.00
24.5	0.66	0.65	0.64	0.63					

Figure 3 WTE conversion table (Bailey, 1998)

Reflection

There are eight bank holidays throughout the year in England. Four of them occur in the Easter season, usually April and May. If staff normally earn extra pay for bank holiday working it is often factored into their total wage, which is then paid in 12 monthly instalments. This means that during the Easter season it can appear that budget is overspent on staff pay.

1. Are there times in your annual budget when you appear to be paying staff more than usual? If so, can you identify why this happens? (See Budget reports.)

Budget for the period

This will be the cumulative (total) budget to date. For example, £1,900 × 8 months = £15,200.

Expenditure for period

The cumulative or total expenditure to date.

Over/under (+/−) variance

Over/under variance is the comparison of the budget to date and the expenditure to date. Overexpenditure is not necessarily a bad thing as there could be a valid reason for it, such as bulk buying that could be accounted for by phasing the budget. On the other hand, underexpenditure is not necessarily a good thing because payment for some goods may not have been completed.

BUSINESS PLANNING

Business planning involves creating a detailed plan for a programme or service and includes the strategy and business goals relating to the provision, expansion or marketing of a product and/or service. A business plan is a financial plan. You may be asked for a business plan when a service is to be introduced or expanded. Business plans do not have to be complex. They are basically an estimate of the amount of money that is needed to achieve a certain service. For example, if you wanted to introduce a nurse-led continence clinic in a day care centre you would need to:

- identify the need for the service;
- state the frequency of the clinic;

- set the goals of the service – for example, the number and throughput of patients, the advantages to patients, etc.
- provide information on the proposed staffing and the required qualifications of staff (for all staff including the records staff and the receptionist, not just nursing staff);
- provide the training costs, if needed;
- identify the specific equipment and supplies needed;
- state how much room is required (if the space needed cannot also be used for another purpose).

BUDGETING TERMINOLOGY

Cash flow

Cash flow is an analysis of expected or actual receipts and payments of cash on a periodic basis.

Depreciation

Depreciation is a financial measure of the wearing out of a capital asset. If an asset costs £40,000 new and lasts four years it will depreciate at the rate of £10,000 a year. Therefore, the asset is worth £20,000 at the beginning of the third year and nothing at the end of the fourth year. However, buildings, which are also capital assets, have a tendency to increase in value over time, though they can also depreciate, particularly if they are purpose built and it is costly to alter them.

Direct costs

Direct costs are those that can be easily identified as belonging to a peculiar cost centre or activity.

Indirect costs

Indirect costs are those that are not easily identified as belonging to a particular cost centre or activity.

Expenditure costs

These are costs that are incurred as a result of expenditure like, for example, cash spending and the interest incurred by spending on credit over a particular time period.

Fixed budget

A fixed budget is one that is unchanging despite changes in activity.

Fixed costs

Fixed costs are total costs that are unchanging with changes in activity levels.

Historically based budgeting

This is a method of drawing up financial plans by applying a consistent formula of increase from one year to the next.

Income

Income is the amount of cash received and the change in the amount of cash owing over a specified period. Money is paid for patient services into a care organisation. Approximately half of the money paid for caring for patients goes for direct care such as nursing and medical staffing. The other half is paid for the support services such as catering, cleaning, administration, etc. (See Figure 4.)

Operating budget

An operating budget is a plan of anticipated activity and the required resources for day-to-day activity within the organisation.

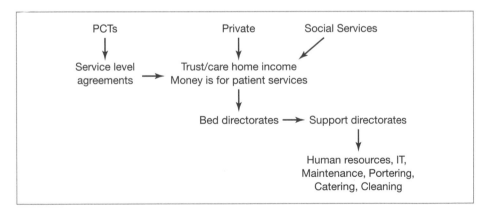

Figure 4 Flow of money into Trusts/care homes

Activity-based budgeting

This is a method of budget setting that 'flexes' the budget in accordance with changes in activity. Therefore, budgets increase with increasing activity and decrease with decreasing activity.

CONTRACTING

Services may be contracted from different purchasers, (see Figure 4). Contracts for service are legal documents so, if the contract is not fulfilled by the supplier, they can be sued in law. When contracting takes place within an organisation such as, for example, the NHS, service level agreements (SLA) are used instead of contracts. For example, a Primary Care Trust (PCT) placing a contract with an NHS Trust will use a SLA. SLAs are not contracts because one part of an organisation cannot sue another part of the same organisation. However, if a large care charity asks a university to supply training, then they would use a contract because the charity is a different organisation. Contracts should include the following features.

Service delivery specifications

- What is to be delivered?
- How much?
- To whom?
- When?
- And where?

Quality standards

- How long should patients wait for treatment?
- What should patients expect when being treated?
- How can patients complain if they are not satisfied?
- Measures for controlling infection outbreaks and treatment.

Information requirements

- Measures of performance, such as the number of patients treated, the number of visits, etc.
- Reporting on a regular basis, for example, monthly reports that are relayed to the purchaser.

Contracts should be feasible; it is pointless agreeing to a contract that cannot be fulfilled. For this reason, front-line managers should be involved in the contracting process as they often have the knowledge necessary to create feasible and relevant contracts.

Key Learning Points

Budgets are controlled by:

- Writing budget reports that clearly present costs and expenditure;
- Business planning when expanding or marketing a service;
- Understanding budgeting terms;
- Writing realistic achievable contracts for suppliers.

Summary of Key Learning Points

The important issues regarding the management of your budget include:

- Being aware of the principles of budgeting – for example, money cannot be spent twice;
- Understanding and applying financial codes and practices relevant to the public domain;
- Having a clear view of what 'value for money' is in relation to your care environment.

Budgeting skills include:

- Understanding how to manage your expenditure;
- Understanding differences in costs (for example, direct and indirect costs) and how to control your costs by controlling expenditure.

Budgets are controlled by:

- Writing budget reports that clearly present costs and expenditure;
- Business planning when expanding or marketing a service;
- Understanding budgeting terms;
- Writing realistic achievable contracts for suppliers.

Case study 1

Mr Robinson was an effective clinical manager in a busy 90-bedded care home but he struggled to understand financial matters. His budget was regularly overspent and he missed deadlines, which put him under pressure when he met with his regional manager. The regional manager was keen to support him and suggested that he spend more time attempting to understand his budgets with advice from the finance team. Despite following these suggestions, the difficulties remained.

During the annual appraisal interview with his home administrator Mrs Patel, it became apparent that while she enjoyed the job and the environment, she lacked stimulation and felt undervalued. She had previously worked in an accounts department and was involved in budget setting.

1. What do you suggest could be done by the manager in these circumstances?
2. What could be the consequences of his actions?

Case study 2

The care of the elderly directorate wards appeared to be overspending on staff wages each month and, as a result, an end-of-year deficit was predicted. Pressure was being placed on the ward managers and the service manager to cut staffing levels. At first it was difficult to determine why the problems were occurring. The ward establishments had been agreed with the finance department when the budget was agreed and there was no overstaffing. A meeting between the service manager and the ward managers revealed that the budget did not take account of the wards being a 24 hour/7 day week service. The money given for staff pay in the budget appeared to be for 9 to 5 coverage. A meeting was called with the finance department, which agreed to rectify the difference. Other issues including the delays in receiving budget reports were discussed and these were also resolved.

1. Do you have an opportunity to discuss budgets with other local managers from your directorate, those in sister homes or with a representative from your finance department?
2. Using your own budget sheets, how would you pick up this type of discrepancy? If you do not know, have a discussion with your manager or your finance department.

Activities

For all of the following activities, if you are not a budget holder then discuss the activity with a colleague who is.

1. Where would you find savings if you were overspent? (See Budgeting Skills.)
2. What are your priorities when organising a budget? (See Definitions and Principles of Budgeting.)
3. How do you balance the different needs within your budget? (See Definitions and Principles of Budgeting.)
4. Check your organisation's written financial practices. Do they give adequate guidance for day-to-day budgeting? (See Budget reports.)
5. What are the key expenditure items in your organisation's budget that relate to quality of care? (See Principles of Budgeting, Chapter 9: Workforce Planning and Skill Mix and Chapter 12: Information and Quality.)
6. What service would you like to introduce into your area? What information would you need in order to complete a business plan? (See Business Planning.)

Chapter 11

Resource management

INTRODUCTION

The topic of resource management will enable you to address National Occupational Standards A4 'Manage activities to meet requirements' and D4 'Provide information to support decision making'.

In this chapter you will:

- consider the broad range of activities involved in resource management;
- understand new developments in staffing and information management;
- consider the complexities involved in equipment costs, including the costs of supplies and drugs;
- be aware of the resource implications in buildings and managing space;
- understand the importance of allocation and time management.

DEFINITIONS AND PRINCIPLES OF RESOURCE MANAGEMENT

Resource management is an essential part of providing quality patient care. It is very important to use resources effectively and efficiently to reduce wastage and avoid inappropriate practice. In the private sector the market is the driving force behind the provision of services and, over the years, there have been attempts to develop scientific means of allocating resources in health and social care organisations. The resources that are required to provide care in all sectors are the same, namely:

- people;
- equipment;
- buildings;
- money;
- information.

All resources have a value, they are constrained and they can be managed. However, there are always cost restraints of some kind. A manager's relationship with their resources will be dependent on the availability of the resource, the source of supply and the amount of money they can access. It is not uncommon for managers to regard only their budget as a resource, due to the emphasis on balancing budgets, forgetting the other factors which should be taken into account. Managers should have the skills and power to enable them to monitor and control the use of the resources for which they are accountable. It is essential to include clinicians in the management of resources, as clinical decisions influence:

- the cost of, for example, drugs, dressings, etc.;
- staffing numbers – the types of patients/clients and their medical and social requirements require accurate resource information.

There is a need in any health and social care service to establish the quality of the service to be delivered, and the costs that are involved in the process of providing that service. Resource management should be a supportive process, underpinned by sound management principles and the professional practice of health care delivery. Management of resources is concerned with all aspects of managing the clinical process and can provide an opportunity to integrate quality of care principles and management, as well as providing a means of communication across managerial and professional boundaries.

Nurses and care managers have to manage:

- budgets (see Chapter 10: Financial Management);
- staff (see also Chapter 9: Workforce Planning and Skill Mix, Chapter 8: The Recruitment and Selection of Staff and Chapter 2: Managing Reflective Practice and Clinical Supervision);
- information (see Chapter 12: Information and Quality Management);
- equipment, including supplies and drugs;
- buildings;
- the process of allocation;
- the time that they have available.

Budgets

Managing budgets in health and social care environments depends largely on decisions made at national level regarding the allocation of resources. Social care environments are very diverse and include nursing homes, residential care, day care, learning disabilities establishments and hospices. The funding of these environments includes a complex mix of government funds, charities and user funding. It is the manager's responsibility to manage consumption and prevent waste (Bryans, 2005).

Staff

The workforce is the most important and the most expensive resource in health and social care environments and is currently undergoing great changes. The Social Care Institute for Excellence is collating and promoting best practice and the General Social Care Council is setting new requirements for training (Batty, 2004). A register is already in existence and social workers and social work students are being registered. Over time social care workers of all levels, from care workers through to directors of social services, will be required to register (General Social Care Council, 2007).

Information

Information is a very important management resource for health and social care staff. There are initiatives underway to develop electronic social care records that mirror the electronic care records in the health service. This initiative is generally run by the local authorities but it is envisaged that the private sector will have access to clients' records (Department of Health, 2007). A recent survey indicates that most local authorities have implemented social care management records but they are very much in the early stages and integration throughout the sector is limited (Department of Health, 2007).

Key Learning Points

When managing resources it is important to realise:

- All resources can be managed but all have cost implications;
- Resource management requires the co-operation of all staff;
- Changes in legislation can have serious implications for resource management.

EQUIPMENT

Managing equipment is an essential aspect of a manager's job. Managers should make sure appropriate equipment is readily available for the tasks to be undertaken, staff are trained to use the equipment and the equipment is serviced at regular intervals.

It is essential that the following factors are taken into consideration in conjunction with clinical requirements when ordering new equipment.

The cost of the equipment

Equipment costs include:

- the initial cost of the equipment;
- the cost of servicing;
- the cost of training staff to use the equipment;
- ongoing consumables;
- the opportunity cost of not buying the equipment;
- the life expectancy of the equipment;
- the cost of storage;
- use with other equipment.

Initial costs can be reduced by negotiating discounts for quantity with manufacturers. Alternatively, expensive equipment such as pressure-relieving mattresses can be hired. While the initial cost of hiring may be lower, if equipment is in regular or constant use, in the long run it can be cheaper to buy equipment. The policy of buying the same make of equipment can reduce training costs and can also decrease the mistakes which can occur if different equipment is purchased.

Servicing equipment

Equipment has to be serviced at regular intervals to ensure that it is in working order. The costs of servicing should be estimated and taken into account when purchasing equipment. Some manufacturers have maintenance courses for organisations and attendance at such courses can reduce servicing costs.

Equipment consumables

The cost of consumables can be considerable. If, for example, equipment is used with disposables, the cost of these should be taken into account. It is

Reflection

It is not usual in the health service for equipment to be bought from charitable donations. Most hospitals now have a policy of ensuring all equipment bought is in accordance with their guidelines after many mistakes were made with syringe drivers. Syringe drivers are electronic syringes which deliver measured doses of drugs over a period of time. Different makes had different gauges and some hospitals had many different makes of driver, which resulted in some patients receiving overdoses. Similar problems were encountered with the original blood glucose monitors used for diabetic patients.

1. How do you ensure that your equipment is used correctly?
2. If a new piece of equipment is introduced into an area, are staff members systematically trained to use it? Or is it a question of leaving the staff in the area to find out how it should be used?

also essential to ensure that attachments for equipment, for example, slings for hoists are sufficient and suitable for all types of patients.

The opportunity cost

It should be possible to estimate the opportunity costs of not buying the equipment. For example, the cost of buying pressure-relieving mattresses can be offset against the cost of treating patients with pressure sores. It can be difficult to make this calculation and there may be no incentive to initiate the process as money spent in one budget may be saved over a period of time, perhaps by another budget holder.

Reflection

Most house holders make an opportunity cost calculation when they insulate their homes. The initial cost can be great, but there will be considerable savings over a period of time that will justify the initial cost. The house holder will be responsible for both cost and savings. In health and social care it can be more difficult to estimate the savings that will occur over a period of time as more variables have to be taken into account (for example, patient condition, etc.) whereas the expenditure itself may all come out of one annual budget.

1. If you had unlimited funds to spend in order to save money in the long run, what cost efficient changes would you try to introduce into your area?
2. Try to calculate the costs versus the savings that could be made and the length of time it will take to justify the expenditure.

Depreciation

Medical equipment often has a life expectancy that should be taken into account at the time of purchase. This life expectancy should be used to estimate the 'book value' of all the equipment you have. This means that if the equipment is new it is worth the purchase price but, if it is a year old, depreciation should be taken into account. For example, if a piece of equipment cost £50,000 and its life expectancy is five years, it will depreciate by £10,000 each year and be worth nothing in six years' time.

Equipment storage

Storage of equipment can often be a difficulty and can have a cost attached. Storage space is rarely taken into account when buildings are constructed or converted, or when equipment is purchased. It is not uncommon to find that if staff members have to walk any distance to obtain equipment, they rarely use it. Large bulky items can also be a fire hazard if stored in a thoroughfare.

Using new equipment with existing equipment

Equipment may also be purchased without taking into consideration how it is used in conjunction with other equipment. For example, hoists may not fit under the beds you are using. Many areas have items of equipment that they are unable to use or that have become obsolete due to the purchase of other equipment.

Reflection

Think about buying a new car. When you drive it off the forecourt it will already have depreciated in value. After one year it will depreciate even further and its second-hand value will have reduced. The same is true for much medical equipment and this should be taken into account because, within a set period, it may need replacing.

1. Look at the equipment in your care environment. How much of it needs replacing now or in the near future? Was this taken into account when purchasing or are you using equipment past its 'sell-by' date as there is no money to replace it?

MANAGING SUPPLIES AND DRUGS

Similar considerations should be taken into account when managing supplies and drugs. It can be more difficult for managers to control budgets in these areas as drugs are prescribed according to medical need, and the supplies of disposable equipment required will be dependent on the clinical condition of the patient. Drug costs can be decreased by the use of generic drugs, the use of alternative suppliers, bulk buying, correct storage and ordering according to usage to eliminate waste.

Medical surgical disposables should also be managed proactively. Supplies should be ordered appropriately. While costs should be taken into consideration, if the supplies cannot be used effectively and efficiently more expensive purchases may save money. Costs can also be decreased by ensuring staff are aware of the price of disposables and by changing the layout of storage areas.

Key Learning Points

Managing the equipment resource includes:

- Being aware of the ongoing costs of maintaining and replacing equipment;
- Having an understanding of the importance of staff training for the correct use of equipment;
- Staff being aware of the price of supplies and drugs.

Reflection

Retailers use a system known as 'just in time' whereby supplies are delivered on a daily basis as required, thus eliminating the need for storage space. An example of this is Marks and Spencer. Many of their shops now have an extra floor. The space that used to be storage at the top of the building is now used as a sales floor. More money is being generated with the same retail space, and the same overheads in the form of rates. There are moves to introduce these ideas into health care, where regular supplies are delivered on a daily basis, eliminating the need for large storage areas. However, managers need to ensure that a method of 'one-off' ordering can be incorporated in such a way that a surge in usage can be overcome and the order list will need to be revised at regular intervals as usage may change over a period.

1. Would this 'just in time' system work in your care environment? On the plus side it could release a lot of storage space but what are the disadvantages?

MANAGING BUILDINGS

Buildings and the space that they provide are often not viewed as a resource. However, space can often be used more effectively.

With the introduction of market forces into all aspects of health and social care, the use of space and the alternative uses for this space should be evaluated on a regular basis. If an area is not being used efficiently, alternative uses should be sought. Space can be used to generate income or improve the services offered.

Reflection

An acute rehabilitation ward in a care of the elderly hospital had some side rooms that were outside the ward on a corridor. While some patients appreciated the privacy this afforded, it was difficult to allocate appropriate patients to these rooms. The rooms could not be allocated to patients who were confused nor to those who needed a lot of assistance as this could mean more than one nurse being away from the ward for a long period. It was decided that a more appropriate use of the rooms was as offices. This enabled the hospital to offer space to speech therapists who, until then, had been based in the community. As a result, speech therapy services were improved for all patients.

1. In your own area is there any space which is underused? If so, what might the alternative uses for the space be? Quality of patient experience and quality of working conditions for staff should also be considered when examining alternative uses.

Opportunity costs in relation to buildings should also be examined. The opportunity cost would be the value of the alternative uses for space if it was not already being used. If a space is in use the opportunity to use it for an alternative purpose is lost so that, for example, if a room is used for storage, it cannot also be used for patient accommodation.

THE PROCESS OF ALLOCATION

The method by which resources are allocated can influence the way in which resources are used. If equipment and/or supplies are stored at a distance from working areas, they may be underused. If unlimited expensive supplies are readily at hand, staff members are unlikely to search out cheaper alternatives. If staff are in plentiful supply, few managers will examine their methods of work and check if unnecessary procedures are being carried out. Alternatively, if there are insufficient employees to undertake the care, staff can become demoralised and sickness rates are likely to increase.

Staff should be aware of the methods used to allocate resources, particularly when they are limited. Staff should also be aware of the way in which requests can be made and of the types of information required to support claims for extra resources.

MANAGING TIME

A resource that is often undervalued is a manager's time. Managers rarely take time into account when planning their day. Time should be used as effectively as possible. It should be remembered that managers are paid not just for what they do, but also for what they know. Time spent in planning is not wasted time. Also, time spent with staff, both individually and in groups, can pay dividends. Management of staff is an essential part of the manager's job. It is important to know staff, be aware of their motivation, their qualifications, experience and developmental needs, and their ambitions. If you have a good knowledge and understanding of staff it may be possible to anticipate problems and prevent serious issues.

Staff are not just numbers in a budget report; they are the most flexible asset of an organisation because they have the potential for development. Therefore, you need to manage the way your staff use their time, as staff time is a very valuable resource. Care organisations are labour intensive, providing care 24 hours a day, seven days a week and 365 days a year. As most care work involves shift work it is necessary that shift patterns ensure sufficient staff and the appropriate skills are available so that you can provide quality care while also making sure staff have a good work/life balance. If managers disregard the latter, it can lead to low morale, high sickness and turnover as well as difficulties in recruiting. Flexible working and job sharing, as well as adherence to working time directives, can all have a favourable influence on the working conditions.

Key Learning Points

Managing and allocating resources includes:

- The effective use of space to generate income and improve services;
- Staff awareness of the cost of resources and the part they play in using resources responsibly;
- The effective and efficient use of the manager's time to plan the use of resources.

Summary of Key Learning Points

When managing resources it is important to realise:

- All resources can be managed but all have cost implications;
- Resource management requires the co-operation of all staff;
- Changes in legislation can have serious implications for resource management.

Managing the equipment resource includes:

- Being aware of the ongoing costs of maintaining and replacing equipment;
- Having an understanding of the importance of staff training for the correct use of equipment;
- Staff being aware of the price of supplies and drugs.

Managing and allocating resources includes:

- The effective use of space to generate income and improve services;
- Staff awareness of the cost of resources and the part they play in using resources responsibly;
- The effective and efficient use of the manager's time to plan the use of resources.

Case study 1

Adam Black is a newly appointed manager of a 40-bedded care home. There has recently been a rise in staff sickness and two members of care staff are on long-term sickness due to back injuries.

1. What information does Adam need to obtain to assure himself that all is being done to avoid any further back injuries?

Case study 2

Ruth Waterson, an experienced home care manager, has been asked to help a friend who has inherited a care home that was owned by her family. The home has had managerial difficulties for some time. It was running at a deficit, had a poor reputation, it was hard to recruit staff and equipment needed updating. A new manager was to be appointed and Ruth has been asked to produce a plan for resources in an attempt to make the home financially viable and able to achieve re-registration.

1. What should be in the plan? List your priorities and give your reasons for them.

Activities

1. Assess the resources available in your care environment, including staff, equipment and buildings.
2. Are you aware of new legislation and initiatives regarding staff registration? What plans are you making in this regard? (See Staff.)
3. Have you heard of electronic social care records? If so, how could your organisation benefit from these? (See Information.)
4. Are you aware of your equipment and replacement costs? (See Equipment.)
5. Have you ever performed an audit regarding the use of space in your care environment? If not, perform one. (See Managing Buildings.)
6. Do you take time during the day to plan the use of resources? (See The Process of Allocation and Managing Time.)

Part Three

Managing Change

Chapter 12

Information and quality management

INTRODUCTION

The topic of information and quality management along with other topics in Part Three will enable you to address National Occupational Standards D4 'Provide information to support decision making' and F3 'Manage continuous quality improvement'. In this chapter you will:

- develop awareness of the ethical and legal principles of information storage and retrieval;
- understand the principles of information management;
- examine a variety of information sources;
- understand the concepts of reliability, validity and sufficiency of information;
- understand the use and application of quantitative and qualitative information;
- develop an awareness of the principles of managing quality;
- understand the use and application of quality circles;
- understand the principles of quality assurance;
- understand the principles and concepts of audit and benchmarking;
- using information sources and assessing quality issues identify the need for change.

INFORMATION MANAGEMENT

Ethical and legal principles for information storage and retrieval

Confidentiality and ethics

All managers must have an awareness and understanding of the law and the ethics of information storage and retrieval. Confidentiality is a very important principle relating to the storage of information. There are moral issues about privacy and also the legal requirements of the Data Protection Act 1998 and the Freedom of Information Act 2002. Information about both acts is available at **www.ico.gov.uk**.

Reflection

When these two acts first came in, staff were not aware of the implications and protested about the extra work safeguarding files and the requirements for giving clients and relatives the information they ask for.

1. Both of these acts apply to the health and social care sector. Are you compliant with them? For example, are clients and relatives aware of their rights under both acts? (See Ethical and legal principles for information storage and retrieval.)

The Department of Health does provide specific guidelines for social services on the Data Protection Act but essentially compliance is the same for all organisations in the public and private sector. For local information about and application of the Data Protection Act the best source of information is your local council website.

The Caldicott Report

The Caldicott Report was commissioned in 1997 to address the implications regarding the confidentiality of Electronic Patient Records (EPR). As with the Data Protection and Freedom of Information Acts, you need to be aware of the main points of the report and the way in which they affect your local practice (Department of Health, 1997). The following website will also be useful: **www.static.oxfordradcliffe.net/confidential/gems/caldrep.pdf**.

The first pilot studies for Electronic Social Care Records (ESCR) are well underway and all workers in the social care sector will need to be aware of the implications. The aim is to have integrated health and social care plans for individuals with long-term conditions by 2008, and for integrated electronic health and social care records for all by 2010 (Department of Health, 2007). The Department of Health issued a circular regarding the implementation of the Caldicott standard into social care settings (Department of Health, 2002) and this can be found at: **www.dh.gov.uk/prod_consum_dh/groups/ dh_digitalassets/@dh/@en/doc-uments/digitalasset/dh_4012213.pdf**.

The implementation of this standard required the appointment of Caldicott Guardians in all social care settings. These Guardians will be responsible for auditing standards of confidentiality for all client-related information.

Information sources

Sources of information include human and technical sources and formal and informal sources. A lot of information is collected in the care setting and this must be managed and rationalised effectively. There are many systems for organising and prioritising information and the choice of a system depends on preference and need, but there are some general principles that apply to all.

Principles of information management

1. Be aware of the information sources available to you, such as clients, relatives, the local authority, the worldwide web.
2. Be aware of the quality and meaning of the information you use. The quality of your decisions depends on the quality of the information and your ability to analyse it.
3. Know how and where to obtain the information you need.
4. Know how to apply the information you use and how to communicate information to others.

Records

Each care environment will decide on what records they will keep and which system they will use to manage these records, but all care organisations will keep records of the following:

- Client information, either as paper records such as care plans and kardex systems or, more commonly nowadays, electronic care plans and files.
- Financial information for records of expenditure, income and staffing.
- Personnel records regarding attendance, performance, sickness, training, etc.
- A daily monitoring system that includes diaries, message systems, emails, contact details for staff, clients and relatives, etc.

We probably pay least attention to the daily record but, in terms of efficiency, it is probably the most important.

> **Reflection**
>
> A local care home purchased a very expensive top-of-the-range electronic record-keeping system but, when visiting students, I found they were keeping parallel written records in notebooks and on scraps of paper as there was always a queue to access the computer. Having spent all their budget on the system, the home could not afford enough monitors to make it accessible to all the staff.
>
> 1. Examine your record-keeping system. What information do you use on a daily basis? How is it recorded and is it accessible to all who need it? (See Information sources.)

Key Learning Points

Managing information requires:

- Knowledge and understanding of the ethical and legal requirements of information management;
- An understanding of the principles of information management;
- An awareness of the importance of accurate and accessible records.

Analysing information

When using information it needs to be examined for:

- reliability;
- validity;
- sufficiency.

Reliability

Before we base major decisions on the information we have found, we need to know that the information is reliable. For example:

- Does the information come from a trustworthy source (for example, a peer-reviewed journal or a published book)?

- Is the information credible and dependable? Is it accurate and does it match your own experience of the issue or topic in question? Would other people agree with your conclusions based on the information you have chosen?
- Is the information applicable and relevant to the issue you are exploring, i.e. is it transferable to your own situation? For example, if you work in a very small care home, would information about a very large care home be applicable and relevant to your own situation?

Validity

We also need to ask ourselves if the information is valid. Is the information really about what it says it is about? Does it really measure what it says it measures? For example, if someone measures a patient's height using an accurate tape measure we can be pretty sure the result they get is going to be valid. However, if you read an article on the declining health of care home residents in the West Midlands you would need to know the definition of 'health' being used by the author and the way the author is measuring the patients' health before you could be sure the information is valid. If the author hasn't provided this information then you would probably question the validity of the article. Of course, validity is not an absolute concept; it is a matter of degree. For example, information about management in a large care home can be valid to the manager of a very small care home, but only to a certain degree. When assessing the validity of a piece of information you need to decide to what degree it is valid in your particular circumstances. There are various ways of assessing whether a piece of information is valid.

- The 'common sense' test – is the information really about what it says it is about? If not, discard it immediately.
- Would the average person (client or fellow professional) be able to understand the information if you gave it to them? Would they agree with you that the information is about what it says it is about? If not, is it really valid and useful to you?

Sufficiency

Finally, before making a decision based on the information you have gathered, you need to be sure you have enough information in order for your decision to be a good one. Generally, a single source of information, not based on any other expertise or research, cannot usually be relied on as a valid basis for a decision.

> ## Reflection
>
> When working in the National Health Service I discharged many clients into the residential care sector. I assumed that the sector required similar information to that required for a transfer to another hospital. However, as I became more aware of the needs of the sector I realised that the information required was quite different.
>
> 1. Exactly what information do you need when a client is admitted? How do you go about getting that information? How do you know that the information you receive is reliable, valid and sufficient? (See Analysing information.)

Qualitative and quantitative information

Some of the information you deal with will be qualitative, that is information relating to or based on feelings or opinions. Other information you deal with will be quantitative, that is information capable of being measured or expressed in numerical terms. Budgeting and financial management is numerical but information about the satisfaction of clients regarding their care is generally based on feelings and opinions. It is important to be aware of the value of both types of information and that reliability, validity and sufficiency relate to both qualitative and quantitative data.

Qualitative information

Opinions, feelings, judgements and description are all included under the general heading of qualitative information. Much of the information you deal with on a day-to-day basis will come under this heading. For example, client notes – 'had a good night', care plans – 'client tends to be tearful in the evenings, reassure', plus the conversations you have throughout the day are all giving and receiving information. We analyse this information every day according to our judgement of its reliability and validity and the trustworthiness of the producer of the information.

One single care plan or report on a client's day may not be a reliable source of information as it may not be a typical day. If a member of staff reports concerns about a client, a review of all the information about that client would be advisable. Their admission information, recent care plans and ongoing monitoring information regarding their diet, medication and daily activities will help decision making about the ongoing care of the client. This assessment should always include talking to the client, their carers and relatives where appropriate. Formal qualitative analysis includes questionnaires, interviews and observation of practice (Thomas *et al*, 2003).

Quantitative information

Other chapters in this book have dealt with quantitative information (see, for example, the chapters on Financial Management and Resource Management). However, we also deal with and make judgements based on quantitative information on a daily basis. A flushed overheated client will have their temperature taken. Clients should be weighed according to a regular schedule and the results acted upon by adjusting the diet. Medication will be given according to prescription. The concepts of reliability, validity and sufficiency also apply to quantitative information. For example, one high temperature may be due to external factors such as hot beverages, but a series of high temperatures should always be acted upon. A sudden rise or fall in weight should be investigated, although it is wise to check the accuracy of the scales before making dramatic changes in diet. Formal quantitative analysis is by experiment or statistical analysis. Audits can be qualitative or quantitative.

Information and quality

Managing quality depends on the ability to manage and analyse information. One of the problems with information is that managers tend to keep it to themselves. In hierarchical organisations information tends to flow from the top to the bottom of the organisation, with the manager in control of what information is released. Team-based organisations tend to share information on an equal basis (Handy, 1999). An important issue is how much information is shared with clients and relatives. It is often the case that organisations where the quality of care is poor will tend to be secretive and, when the quality of care is good, staff are usually willing to share information with clients, colleagues and relatives.

Key Learning Points

Analysing and applying information requires:

- An understanding of what makes information reliable, valid and sufficient and therefore usable in practice;
- Being aware of the differences between qualitative and quantitative information;
- Being aware of the links between information and quality.

MANAGING QUALITY

The characteristics of quality

Quality is not an optional extra in care settings; it is an essential wherever care is provided to clients or patients (Gould and Merrett, 1992). Quality in health care is difficult for the public to understand because health care is complex:

- Systems of care tend to be paternalistic in that staff tell patients what patients will get.
- Consumerism plays a part, in that the public's perception of quality may not relate to a monetary or statistical value.
- Quality is subjective, i.e. it is not an absolute and perceptions will vary.
- The quality of care is not solely about the outcome, it is also about the way in which care is delivered.
- The way in which patients perceive quality is also a key issue.

Reflection

Most people know what to expect when buying a jumper – you can tell a good-quality one from one that is not. I was asked to be an expert witness for a hospital patient who had sustained a fractured leg after a fall. Before reading the solicitor's letter I had come across a post-operative picture of the patient's leg and I had thought that it was a neat scar given that the patient was over 80. The solicitor's letter read: 'This patient has been left with a horrendous scar.' It was evident that my perception as a nurse, who had worked in orthopaedics, was very different from that of a lay solicitor.

1. How do your clients and their relatives perceive the quality of care in your organisation? (See Managing Quality.)

Quality in care also includes intangibles such as:

- access to services;
- the relevance of care to the needs of patients;
- equity for all;
- the effectiveness of care;
- social acceptability, which is changeable over time;
- efficiency and economy.

A quality service

A quality service:

- needs to be well-designed;

- needs to provide satisfaction;
- does not make mistakes as these have a cost implication for an organisation – fewer mistakes saves money.

What is quality?

Is quality the overall character of the performance, or compliance in fulfilling specified norms, or is it consistency in meeting a standard nearly all the time?

Quality features

Is there a consensus on:

- the parameters and standards of quality?
- the ways these can be achieved?
- the level at which they should be achieved?
- the priorities?
- how much weight should be given to the different practices involved?

While it is extremely difficult to state exactly what is meant by 'good quality', experienced staff should know what poor quality is and recognise good quality when it occurs. There is a tendency to use numbers wherever possible in order to provide a standard of measurement and to allow for ease of comparison. However, this can mean that league tables and numbers may be used even when inappropriate. Remember that the selection of quality criteria is a key act of leadership and the principal spur to quality is staff motivation.

Reflection

The Patients Charter of 1991 was a good example of creating supposed quality standards which did not necessarily result in a quality service. For example, the maximum time a patient should wait to be seen in Out Patients (OP), after an appointment time, was 30 minutes. To ensure this was achieved, managers had to take note of the times when patients were seen. I was responsible, as a manager, for providing these figures. We had a very large surgery clinic that had a very quick throughput. Patients appeared, on average, to spend only two minutes with the consultant and the figures for the clinic were good. However, some patients in the clinic were being told that they had cancer, and yet they also appeared to be spending the average amount of time with the doctor. From my point of view this was not a quality service, yet it fulfilled the criteria to which we had to adhere.

1. Reflect on your own practice. How do you judge quality of care? List the ways you do this. Are these ways based on statutory requirements or your own personal standards?

Models and theories of quality

Quality circles

Quality circles originated in the US in the 1950s. The ideas were then imported into Japan and 30 years later, re-exported to the US. Prior to the Second World War, any goods stamped with 'Made in Japan' were internationally considered of poor quality. However, in the 1950s the Japanese realised that, in order to compete internationally, they had to improve their quality of output. They were aware that America, despite its industrial prowess, had a quality problem, as many American bombs dropped on Japan during the war had failed to explode. William Deming advocated that quality had to be incorporated systematically into the whole of an industrial process and spent two decades after the war teaching these methods to the Japanese. Thirty years later, Europe and the US re-imported the ideas, having identified them as a major factor in Japanese industrial success.

Quality circles are groups of workers who meet on a regular basis to discuss and analyse problems, suggest solutions and take appropriate action regarding quality issues in their areas of responsibility. Poor quality has both tangible and intangible costs attached for care organisations, and for clients and patients. Organisations that improve quality can cut costs by up to 50 per cent while also improving productivity and increasing customer satisfaction.

The quality process consists of three interrelated activities: planning; improvement and control (Juran Institute, 1993) (see Figures 1 and 2). The ultimate goal of the quality process is perfection or zero deficit.

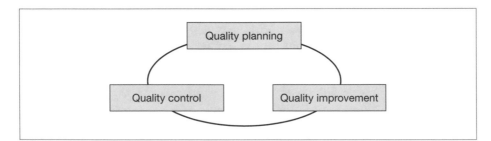

Figure 1 Juran trilogy of total quality management (adapted from Juran Institute, 1993)

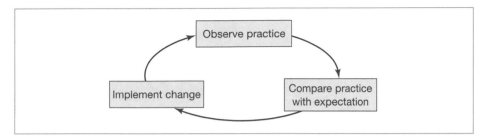

Figure 2 Quality in action: the quality circle (Gould and Merrett, 1992, p. 4)

Reflection

Remember your first car? One of my first cars was an old VW Beetle, but it had heating! The heating system was fairly primitive. Your left foot was very warm (as this was where the hot air entered the car) and the rest of the car was warmish. At the time heating was an innovation. Today, at the very least, you would expect an efficient whole-car heating system, a heated back window, and heated seats in a new car. Customers these days have higher expectations; they are better educated and live life at a faster pace.

1. Reflect on the changes that have occurred in the service you give to your clients/residents. Were these proactive changes or the result of pressure from consumers? List any means you have of regularly examining the quality of your service? Does the process work? If not, why not? (See Managing Quality.)

Quality planning

Quality planning should be a team effort and involve organisational time and resources. If deficiencies or problems can be overcome the first time they occur, up to 20 per cent of costs can be reduced. Goals need to be set, measurement criteria established and monitoring methods planned. Richards and Heginbotham's (1992) language of quality includes:

- Inspection quality:
  o monitoring;
  o check lists.
- Accreditation quality:
  o standards;
  o volume.
- Management quality:
  o performance review;
  o service management;
  o case management.

- Clinician quality:
  o good practice;
  o clinical audit;
  o care;
  o effectiveness.

Quality assurance

Quality assurance carries a commitment to respond positively to results from an evaluation or an assessment. It is not a wish list; action must be taken to modify practice wherever necessary. Expectation of practice should be expressed in a format of measurable standards; practices which do not meet standards have to be improved. Assessments should be carried out at regular intervals as an integrated part of practice. Improving quality can also save money. Up to 20 per cent of costs in health care can be spent attempting to remedy poor quality, such as finding patients' notes. If everything is correct first time, these costs can be avoided (see Figure 3) (Juran Institute, 1993).

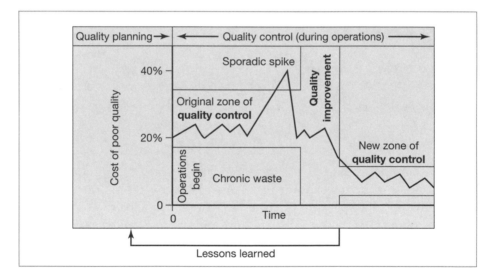

Figure 3 Managing the cost of poor-quality practices (Juran Institute, 1993, p. 18)

Setting standards

Formal standards are a measure of how well any aspect of care should be managed and, where possible, should be based on the evidence of research. Standards can be set by external bodies, such as government, professional bodies and research-based organisations. Internally, they can be set by staff, based on their view of what constitutes best practice.

Reflection

An example of a standard:

Monitoring complaints – all letters received must be acknowledged within five working days. All letters received must be recorded. All complaints must be investigated by the manager of the area concerned within 21 working days if possible. A reply should be sent within 28 working days. Total complaints must be monitored, recorded and collated, analysed and fed back to staff quarterly.

1. Analyse your methods of setting standards. Are the standards appropriate and workable? If not, why not? How could they be improved?

Audit

The word 'audit' originates in the Latin word *auditas* which means a hearing. It was originally used in situations where the facts and arguments about an issue were heard in order to determine the truth. Traditionally it has been used for financial accounts. Nursing audits have been in use since the 1950s and are a means of 'exercising assurance' on the quality of care. Medical audits originated in the US in 1900, and have since been incorporated into clinical governance as clinical audit. Clinical audit involves input from all professionals involved in clinical care. Clinical audit may be seen as a cycle of six stages (see Figure 4).

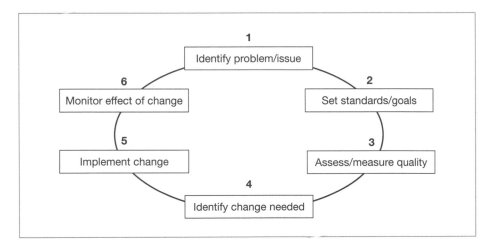

Figure 4 The clinical audit cycle (Kogan and Redfern, 1995, p. 42)

Audit information can be collected on present standards, either qualitatively or quantitatively, using present data, retrospective data or prospective information. It can be collected from all involved in the care process including the clients, residents or patients and their relatives. Various formats such as questionnaires, forms and interviews can be used, and the information collated is then analysed and any problems or issues identified. You need not carry out a formal audit as part of a quality process, but the issues still need to be identified and addressed.

Monitoring

Once specific standards are set it is relatively easy to monitor practice and compare this to the standards. If the standards are not being achieved, the changes required should be identified and carried out and the standard re-monitored.

Problems in attempting to improve quality

The following problems can occur when you are trying to improve quality:

- A lack of constancy of purpose as a result of changing goals.
- Emphasis on short-term gains – quality takes time to achieve.
- Using figures alone, not qualitative data, to illustrate quality.
- It has been calculated that 85 per cent of quality problems in organisations are due to system failures, and only 15 per cent can be attributed to people.

Questions to be asked when examining quality

You need to ask yourself the following questions when you are examining quality:

- What is your aim?
- Who are your customers?
- What do you want your organisation to become as far as quality is concerned?
- How are you going to get there?
- What are the barriers?
- How will you know you are making progress?
- What will be your principal processes?
- What is most in need of improvement?

Benchmarking

An alternative to setting standards is to use benchmarking. This is where your performance is compared with that from other successful organisations. This prevents unrealistically high or unnecessarily low standards from being set. Benchmarking tools are available for aspects of basic care from the Department of Health (2001). The process of benchmarking is shown in Figure 5. If staff are unused to setting standards, it is helpful to use this process. Statements of care can be made as in Figure 6, and compared with practice. This process can also be used in management.

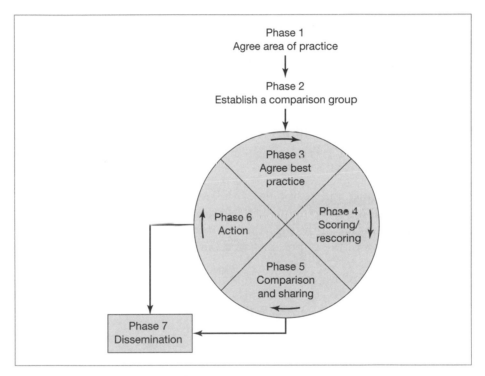

Figure 5 The benchmarking process (Department of Health, 2001)

Worst practice statement	Statements of practice that step towards best practice			Best practice statement
E	D	C	B	A

Figure 6 Statements of care

To achieve improvements in quality, it is helpful if the following factors are taken into account:

- All decisions must be based on facts.
- The people who know the work the best are those who should perform it.

- Groups working in teams are more successful than individuals alone.
- Teams need to be trained in structured problem solving.
- Knowledge of how to conduct meetings assists in the process.
- It is helpful to display information and feedback graphically as this supports different learning styles.

Key Learning Points

Improving the quality of care requires:

- An understanding of models and theories of quality assurance;
- An understanding of the principles of quality planning;
- Knowing how to set standards of care;
- An understanding of the principles of audit and benchmarking.

Summary of Key Learning Points

Managing information requires:

- Knowledge and understanding of the ethical and legal requirements of information management;
- An understanding of the principles of information management;
- An awareness of the importance of accurate and accessible records.

Analysing and applying information requires:

- An understanding of what makes information reliable, valid and sufficient and therefore usable in practice;
- Being aware of the differences between qualitative and quantitative information;
- Being aware of the links between information and quality.

Managing quality requires:

- An understanding of the characteristics of quality;
- Being aware of the intangible elements of quality care;
- An understanding of the features of quality.

Improving the quality of care requires:

- An understanding of models and theories of quality assurance;
- An understanding of the principles of quality planning;
- Knowing how to set standards of care;
- An understanding of the principles of audit and benchmarking.

Case study 1

Mrs Sally Smith is an experienced care home manager who is excellent at managing the staff. She had a good assistant who used to take care of the paperwork but the assistant has left. Sally is now feeling overwhelmed by the amount of information she has to manage.

1. What can Sally do to manage the information in a way that keeps everything running smoothly?
2. If Sally gets a new assistant, how can she ensure that things are not thrown into chaos again?

Case study 2

Mr John Hamilton has recently been appointed assistant manager of a large residential nursing home. There have been problems of quality in patient care, in part due to staff shortages and the use of agency care staff. John has been given the task of putting measures in place to ensure the quality of care improves despite the staff shortages.

1. What measures could be useful to ensure a consistent good quality of care is achieved?
2. What factors should be taken into account when introducing new measures?

Activities

1. Find out what your local council is doing with regard to the Data Protection and Freedom of Information acts. Do you have copies of locally available leaflets on data protection and freedom of information? (See Ethical and legal principles of information storage and retrieval.)
2. Who is your Caldicott Guardian? Talk to them if possible and find out what their view of their role is. (See The Caldicott Report.)
3. Reflect on your own organisation. List the good-quality features and any deficiencies you feel there are in the quality of care that your organisation offers clients. Do the same for a service that you receive from others in your organisation. (See The characteristics of quality.)
4. Do you regularly audit your services? If not, how do you ensure that you have a quality service? How do you deal with complaints, mistakes or 'near misses'? (See Audit.)

Chapter 13

The management of change

INTRODUCTION

The topic of the management of change will enable you to address National Occupational Standards F3 'Manage continuous quality improvement', A4 'Contribute to improvements at work' and SNH4U1 'Develop programmes, projects and plans'. In this chapter you will:

- consider definitions of change and reflect on the changes in your working life;
- gain an understanding of different types of change and the effect on the organisation;
- understand and apply theories of change;
- diagnose the need for change and analyse the processes involved;
- consider the factors involved in managing change;
- gain an understanding of the relationship between power and change;
- gain an awareness of the factors that cause resistance to change.

DEFINITIONS OF CHANGE

While the word 'change' means 'to make or become different', this statement does not take into account the complexities of the concept in management terms and it can be difficult to state exactly what is meant by change. Change will depend on the context in which it occurs and the control that is exercised. Alvin Toffler (1970) in *Future Shock* argued that the rate of change is out of control, and that this has psychological implications. There is a limit to the amount of change that humans can handle but change is also necessary for survival (Huczynski and Buchanan, 2001, p. 521). In service industries technological change together with 'consumerism' and instant feedback has intensified the need for change and survival. Change is essential for the survival of organisations and managers can be the agents for this change.

> ## Reflection
>
> Consider the external and internal factors in the list below and reflect on the changes that have occurred within your workplace in the last year.
>
> - External:
>   o technology – materials;
>   o customers' tastes;
>   o competitors' activities;
>   o legislation;
>   o social and/or cultural values;
>   o changing economic circumstances.
> - Internal:
>   o job design/skill requirements;
>   o the layout of new buildings;
>   o the allocation of responsibilities.

Many changes both at work and in the home have been welcomed. For example, homes are more comfortable than they were 40 years ago with central heating and more efficient appliances.

Types of change

Routine change

The aim of routine change is to maintain a steady state and can just be day-to-day problem solving. This is only recognised as a change by those who have been absent when the change occurred, such as a change in the type of continence sheets supplied. It can be major or extensive, but it is not designed to transform or radically change an organisation. For example, refurbishing a kitchen is a change but it does not alter the nature and/or basic use of the kitchen.

Induced and planned change

Within an organisation planned change is fairly comfortable for all concerned because it is incremental. However, planned change does require energy and active management as it can be a long process. Individuals may need to be coached over a period of time and managers must be committed to the process for it to succeed.

Innovative change

Innovative change can occur as a result of trial and error, for example, experimenting with changing shift patterns. If staff members are creative and/or if incentives are offered this can produce innovative change. However, often a task force or an expert is assigned to bring about change. Innovative change is encouraged when managers are professionally trained, have high job satisfaction, power is devolved and quality rather than quantity is encouraged. On the other hand, recruiters tend to recruit people like themselves and bureaucratic organisations tend to attract individuals that dislike change (Handy, 1993). People who like change and creative thinking rarely opt to work in a bureaucracy because they become frustrated at the speed of change. This can be a problem for bureaucracies.

Crisis change

This type of change is the least desirable and most uncomfortable for all involved. Plans can be made for when a crisis happens, for example, planning in case of a fire, and individuals will allow their behaviour to be radically changed while the crisis is in process. A crisis can be turned into a success, but this type of change should not be needed unless there is an unexpected deviation like a power cut, war or an accident.

Key Learning Points

Understanding the effects of change requires awareness of:

- The context of the change;
- The type of change.

THEORIES OF CHANGE

The stages of change (see Figure 1) were first described by Lewin (1951). These are:

1. Unfreezing – a problem is perceived and there is a desire for change;
2. Moving – change occurs and the activities associated with change take place;
3. Refreezing – people adapt to the change.

Most change is not linear, i.e. it does not go in a straight line. Change takes time and has 'knock-on effects'. As it involves people and structures, change often reflects the idiosyncratic nature of the people who are involved.

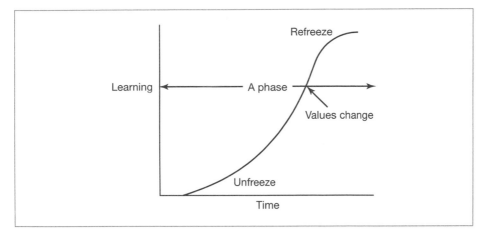

Figure 1 The learning curve (Lewin, 1951 in Hunt, 1986, p. 264)

Reflection

Think about the practical skills you have learned such as driving, playing computer games and giving an injection. It can take time to master the initial skill, and then it can appear that there is no improvement for a time. If the learner persists, mastery is eventually gained. This is easily illustrated by the scores obtained when learning computer games. Also once you have learned a particular type of computer game, other similar games are much easier as learning is transferable.

Lippett (1973) who worked with Lewin (1951) added some detail to the theory of change by identifying activities that could help to move the change agent through the stages of Lewin's theory (see Figure 2). These activities will be familiar to health and social care workers as they are the theory behind the care planning process that we use in individualised care. Every health and social care worker using care planning should be acting as a change agent.

Lewin	Lippett
Unfreezing	Awareness, analysis, assessment. Devise change objectives which should be observable, measurable, timed.
Moving	Choosing a change agent to 'manage' the change. Implement step-by-step change strategies.
Refreezing	Maintenance of change. Terminate helping relationships.

Figure 2 Moving through the change process (Lippett, 1973)

Lewin's theory was intended to be used in practice and has been well tested in many different situations.

Unfreezing/assessment

This part of the cycle of change refers to the process of identifying what needs to be changed and devising a practical plan of action. An assessment of current practice should be carried out and initial objectives set for change. This should be done in the context of both human and financial resources.

Moving/planning

At this stage a 'change agent' should be identified. The manager may fulfil this role themselves or they may delegate it to a suitable senior member of staff. Change agents require authority and the ability to make decisions. The change agent will manage the change by implementing strategies based on the objectives.

Refreezing/evaluating

When the change is implemented it needs to be maintained so that it becomes part of normal everyday practice. The change agent may be able to withdraw at this point but careful evaluation is needed to ensure that withdrawal will not lead to the collapse of the change.

DIAGNOSING THE NEED FOR CHANGE

Iles (1997) states that it is not the role of managers to solve problems, but that they should facilitate a solution to the problem. This is particularly relevant in the management of change. If staff have input in the change process, they are more likely to support the change. It is important to avoid inappropriate change and in order to do this, it is necessary to ensure that the key issues in an organisation are diagnosed correctly. A SWOT analysis is often carried out as part of the diagnosis. SWOT stands for:

S = Strengths;
W = Weaknesses;
O = Opportunities;
T = Threats.

The SWOT analysis should not just consist of a list of facts but should be an analysis of the situation (Iles, 1997).

Reflection

An expansion in the size of your care home may be an opportunity for the organisation because it will be more financially secure if the beds are full. It can also be a threat if it is difficult to recruit suitable staff. This is because patients may not be admitted, but there will still be increased overhead costs and perhaps a mortgage to pay.

1. Attempt to carry out a SWOT analysis of your own organisation/department. Remember that Strengths can also be Weaknesses and Opportunities can also be Threats.

Steps in the analysis process

1. Data collection. It is important that those who will be involved in any change participate in data collection.
2. Define the change.
3. Diagnosis and identification of likely effects of change.
4. Plan.
5. Action.
6. Consolidation of change. Constant change can be frustrating and change takes time. Without consolidation, behaviour may revert and the change may be lost.
7. Evaluation of the change. This rarely takes place in organisations, with the result that any untoward effects of change are often overlooked. The implications of the benefits or risks of a change process are often not analysed or evaluated. It may be difficult to understand exactly what the implications of change will be, prior to a change.

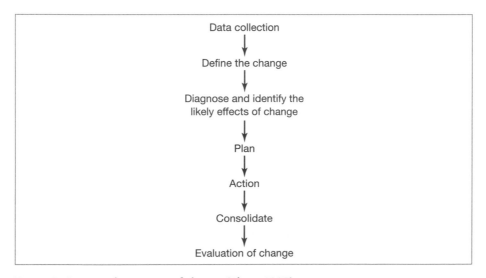

Figure 3 Steps in the process of change (Plant, 1995)

> **Key Learning Points**
>
> The change process requires:
>
> • The ability to analyse factors involved in the change;
> • The avoidance of inappropriate change;
> • The ability to achieve the active involvement of staff in change.

MANAGING CHANGE

It is vital that managers manage the process of change, as illustrated in Figure 4. All staff involved in the change should be approached as early as possible. If news about an impending change is first obtained via the local 'grapevine' it is liable to cause resentment. If there is likely to be a change, then managers should be proactive in providing help. One important question should always be asked: 'do we have the resources in both staff and equipment to implement this change successfully?' It is also important to avoid over organising when managing change. Unexpected events can occur and staff can be encouraged to solve any ensuing problems. Staff involvement and ownership of all stages in the process increases the chances of success.

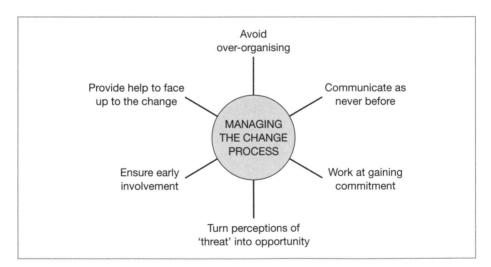

Figure 4 Six key activities for successful implementation of change (Plant, 1995, p. 32)

The commitment of the workforce to change must be obtained and it is essential to communicate consistently throughout the process. Rumours spread more quickly than correct information so it is very important to ensure that reliable information is readily available. Perceptions of threats resulting from change can be turned into opportunities. For example, lack of jobs in one area can mean an opportunity to consider an alternative career move.

It is important that managers are aware of the relationships in an organisation which can influence the process of change, as illustrated in Figure 5. These relationships should be analysed. It is evident that the winners are more likely to embrace a change. The losers should be sought out and involved in the process and perhaps helped specifically with the change.

Reflection

When I was working as a service manager there were strategic plans in place to close a small hospital and transfer all the acute care of the elderly rehabilitation services to the main hospital. It was essential to ensure that the staff who had chosen to work in rehabilitation were able to make the change. The numbers of beds and therefore the number of staff were likely to be reduced in the move. Two years before the move, staff were provided with opportunities to attend courses and encouraged to update their knowledge and skills.

1. Reflect on the changes that you have experienced at work. Did the management attempt to help and support those who may be adversely affected by the change? If not, what effect did this have on the workforce?

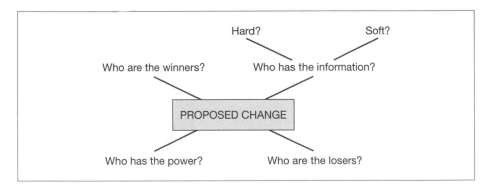

Figure 5 Key relationship mapping (Plant, 1995, p. 24)

While staff will change if their survival is threatened, an imposed change is less likely to be successful in the long term, as shown in Figure 6. It may be time consuming to involve staff, but any changes made are more likely to be successful if members of staff are committed.

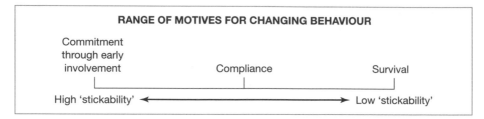

Figure 6 The likelihood of long-term behaviour change (Plant, 1995, p. 23)

Key Learning Points

Managing change requires:

- A knowledge of the key activities for implementing change;
- An awareness of the relationships affecting the change process;
- Understanding the motives for change.

POWER AND CHANGE

Etzioni's Theory of Power

Power	Responses
Coercive	Alienation
Remunerative	Calculating
Normative	Moral

(Etzioni, 1964)

The sociologist Amitai Etzioni worked on power and change for many years and his compliance theory of how power works is still in current use in many organisations. The core of the theory is that change requires power and the type of power that is used will affect the response and therefore the chances of the change succeeding.

Coercive power

Coercive power leads to rapid change. If the consequences of not changing are dismissal or demotion the change will normally take place but the change will be reluctant and often imperfectly implemented as the employees feel alienated and unengaged in the change. There is also the risk that those staff that can leave, will leave.

Remunerative power

Remunerative power means that, if the manager can find the right level and kind of incentive, then staff will change their working practices. Small changes may only require small incentives, such as management approval and a good performance review. If you require staff to make a large change, such as implementing clinical supervision, the incentive may need to be greater: for example, a grade enhancement for those prepared to be clinical supervisors. However the response to remunerative power is calculating. If the member of staff is not convinced that the change is worthwhile their involvement will be superficial and they will not be fully involved in the change. For example, if a short-term bonus is given to encourage change and then it is withdrawn the change will quickly cease to be practised as staff will calculate that it is not worth their while to continue.

Normative power

Etzioni regarded normative power as the key power as it enables communities and organisations to work. If members of staff are involved in the change and agree with the change they will participate willingly without need of force or reward. The response to this power is moral: 'I agree with this as it is for my and others' benefit therefore, I will be fully involved in the change'. If you can achieve a moral response the change in practice will be permanent and become part of normal behaviour. If you cannot evoke a moral response the change will only be maintained by constant vigilance and threats of disciplinary action or expensive incentives.

Using power to change practice

Managers need to understand the power they have to change their organisation and the limits and ethical use of that power. Managers should also be aware of the need for personal change where necessary. Coercive power should be used reluctantly but it may be necessary if clients are being endangered by unsafe practice, for example, care workers failing to wash their hands or failing to cater for clients' basic hygiene needs. Education and support should be used in conjunction with coercive power to assist practice changes and enable changes to be internalised. Alternatively, incentives can be used ethically as levers for change. However, staff have also to be convinced of the efficacy of the change for change to occur successfully. Gaining consensual agreement for change takes time, but the change should be permanent and remains in place when the management changes and when new staff arrive, as the change is presented to them as normal practice.

Key Learning Points

Implementing change requires:

- An understanding of the nature of power;
- An understanding of our own sources of power;
- Using power appropriately and constructively.

Reflection

I have performed this exercise with many groups and the outcome is always the same. I ask the following two questions:

1. Have you ever deliberately parked illegally?
2. Have you ever deliberately failed to stop at a zebra crossing when someone is standing on the kerb?

The majority of the group, sometimes 100 per cent, say 'yes' to the first question and express very little contrition. A very small minority say 'yes' to the second question and most of these are embarrassed and ashamed. The first activity is illegal and subject to a fine so we do not do it when the parking wardens are out. The second activity is only illegal if someone is on the crossing and endangered. Not stopping when someone is on the kerb attracts no penalty except for guilt. As a society we have a collective agreement to stop at zebra crossings and our response is moral and very powerful.

1. Have you ever done more work than is strictly required by your contract when there is no possibility of a penalty if you don't? Why do you do this?

RESISTANCE TO CHANGE

Resistance to change is often an attempt by staff to retain the 'status quo'. Many people do not like change and if there have been many recent changes, some find it very difficult to cope. Resistance can take the form of minimal contributions, indifference, apathy, or personal withdrawal, and sometimes even active resistance can occur. There is a tendency to view resistance as negative, but it can be healthy. Not all change is positive and resistance can lead to a review of the objectives of change and the methods used. Resistance can be due to ignorance, anxiety about change, guilt, rejection or loss of power. 'Political' games can also influence staff. It should be remembered that change will often take much longer than anticipated. It can take time for staff to adapt but it is better to take the time to gain support for change as the change.

Reflection

I was a ward sister when the 'nursing process' was implemented. We all agreed with the concept of 'individualised care' that it was supposed to encourage but we disliked writing care plans as they were perceived as time consuming and difficult. The ward nurses happily switched to caring for groups of clients rather than carrying out tasks for the whole ward but they could not and/or/ would not fill in the care plans correctly. This was in the 1980s but I recently read a management project where the nursing home manager was experiencing exactly the same thing.

1. Should we give up on a change that is self-evidently not working or keep trying to find a solution that is acceptable to all?

Summary of Key Learning Points

Understanding the effects of change requires awareness of:

- The context of the change;
- The type of change.

The change process requires:

- The ability to analyse the factors involved in the change;
- The avoidance of inappropriate change;
- The ability to achieve the active involvement of staff in change.

Managing change requires:

- A knowledge of the key activities for implementing change;
- An awareness of the relationships affecting the change process;
- Understanding the motives for change.

Implementing change requires:

- An understanding of the nature of power;
- An understanding of our own sources of power;
- Using power appropriately and constructively.

Case study 1

The owners of the residential care home where you work have decided to increase the number of beds, and take short-stay convalescent patients as well as long-term residents. It is envisaged that most of the new patients will be day surgery patients, who if they had assistance at home, would have been directly discharged home. As a manager you have been asked to ensure that the staff will be able to care for these types of patients. Many of the staff have worked at the home for some time, and while there has been an ongoing staff development programme, some have never worked in the acute area and others have had little experience with day surgery.

1. How would you undertake the change process in this organisation?
2. Make a plan for change that includes assessment, objectives, strategies and evaluation.

Case study 2

Riverside View is a large residential home with nursing beds and it employs a large number of staff. The home is overspent on its staff budget and this is being addressed by the home manager. She has come up with several ideas but the most cost effective and easiest to implement is a change in the number of hours that staff work. Currently the working day is between 7 a.m. and 9:30 p.m. Many of the competitor homes operate a working day of 8 a.m. to 8 p.m. In practice this means that the home could cut staffing levels to the night ratio for an extra two and a half hours a day. This means saving 84 hours of staff time a week, resulting in savings of over £20,000 a year. This will make up most of the current overspend on staffing. This means the night staff will need to work an extra two hours a night but they will have to work two fewer nights a week in each four-week pay period. The manager initially discusses the problem with her management team and asks them to investigate as to how this will fit in with people's current contracted hours and daily nursing practices such as handover times.

The manager also contacts CSCI and the local authority which purchases most of their beds. She plans meetings with the staff to start the discussion process and decides to meet with the night staff first, as they are the most likely to object to the change. The area manager sees the figures and says this has to be done regardless of how unpopular it may be.

1. Reflecting on this chapter, how would you manage this change?
2. What might the manager do to encourage the staff to see this as a necessary and beneficial change?

Activities

1. Reflect on the way in which change occurs in your organisation. What is the most common type of change? Is innovation encouraged? (See Types of Change.)
2. Reflect on the last change you were involved in, in your organisation. Was it a successful process? If so, why? If there was resistance, what form did it take? (See Diagnosing the Need for Change and Steps in the Process Analysis.)
3. What power do you have to change things in your organisation? Reflect on an area of practice where you would like to introduce change. How could you use your power? (See Power and Change, Using power to change practice and Resistance to change.)

Chapter 14

Negotiation and conflict

INTRODUCTION

The topic of negotiation and conflict will enable you to address National Occupational Standard C13 'Manage the performance of teams and individuals'. In this chapter you will:

- gain an understanding of the sources of conflict within organisations;
- examine strategies for managing conflict;
- gain an understanding of the processes involved in negotiation;
- gain an understanding of the stages of negotiation;
- examine the role of the manager as an arbitrator;
- become aware of the principles and processes involved in dealing with complaints.

CONFLICT

Conflict can exist whenever individual or group interests diverge within organisations, or when an organisation's values or goals are opposed to those of the people who work for it. Conflict is always likely to arise and it is a managerial job to resolve conflict and ensure that it is not a destructive force within an organisation. While it is tempting to avoid confronting situations in which conflict is likely, it is poor management practice not to attempt to resolve issues.

Conflict, and the way it arises and is resolved, is related to the source of power in an organisation and any external influences on that power. It also relates to the ways in which individual managers use their power. Arbitrary and excessive use of power can lead to defiance as this is perceived as the subordinate's only choice. Power can be subtle and complex varying over time between similar organisations and within an organisation. It can be predictable and conventional, or it can be related to other factors such as the possession of information. Conflict can arise from:

- a clash of powerful personalities;
- uncertainty in the face of change;
- management versus professional/care considerations.

Effective management is reliant on:

- a knowledge of the sources of power in an organisation;
- persuading people of the need for change and involving them in the process;
- negotiation and mediation for the resolution of conflict.

Sources of power within organisations include:

- formal authority;
- control of scarce resources;
- the possession of information;
- the possession of special expertise;
- the ability to cope with uncertainty;
- the command of strong networks;
- being a member of the dominant culture;
- the ability to reward or punish.

Reflection

A ward manager was attempting to change the attitudes of her staff. Previously the ward had been a long-term elderly care ward, but now the patients were to be rehabilitated. This meant that patients were to be encouraged to carry out their own activities of daily living with assistance. Most of her staff approved of the changes, but two of her health care assistants (HCAs) (who liked to work together) were opposed to them and tended to obstruct the changes. The ward manager discussed the matter with her manager and one of the HCAs was moved to another ward. The move also enabled both the HCAs to undertake NVQ training, which was difficult when they were on the same ward and required the same time off. The changes in the methods of care went ahead and other changes were planned and implemented, ensuring that the ward gained a reputation for being progressive.

1. Who has the power in your organisation? Do they have formal authority? If not, what is their source of power? (See Conflict and Chapter 13: The Management of Change.)

Activity

Using Figure 1 below as a framework, reflect on how you normally deal with a situation that is likely to be confrontational, for example, a staff member who appears to be absent from work but is not sick, or a staff member who is not 'pulling their weight'.

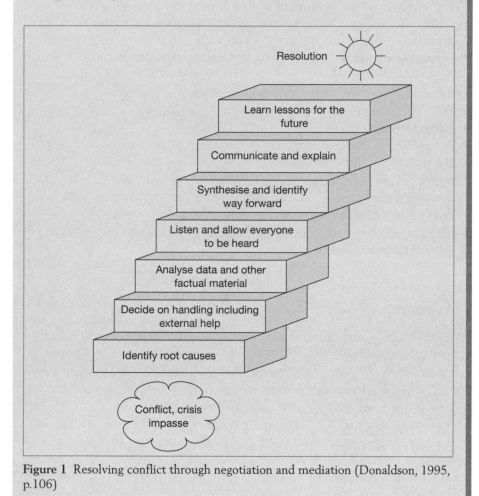

Figure 1 Resolving conflict through negotiation and mediation (Donaldson, 1995, p.106)

Key Learning Points

When dealing with conflict it is important to understand:

- The sources of conflict;
- The sources of power within the organisation;
- The management of confrontations.

NEGOTIATION

You will have been involved in negotiations, whether it was when you were buying a car, a house, or just bargaining on holiday or at the boot fair. In management the ability to negotiate is essential as it can often help you to avoid a conflict situation that can be an unhappy situation for all. At the end of a negotiation, both parties should be satisfied that an appropriate deal has been struck – a win-win situation. In any negotiation there should be an emphasis on the common ground, with a willingness both to relate to the concerns of the other side and to compromise. Negotiating is a complex process, during which:

- the concerns of both sides should be identified (usually through questioning);
- the terms and conditions of a deal should be arranged and agreed;
- there must be a willingness to compromise;
- both sides should relate to the concerns of other side.

Negotiation requires preparation. Different variables, such as the people involved, the objectives and the structure of the negotiating process, have to be taken into account and considered. It should also be remembered that in most instances, there will still be a relationship with the other party at the end of the negotiation and bad feeling should be avoided.

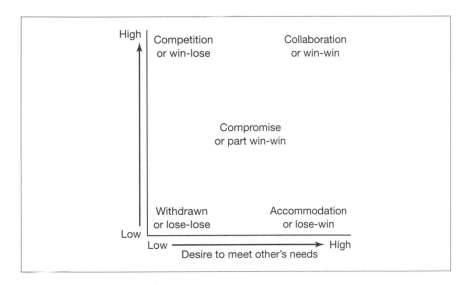

Figure 2 The five behaviours available to parties involved in a conflict (Iles, 1997, p. 31)

How individuals behave in a negotiation depends on how much they want to meet their own needs and how much they want the other party's needs to be met. This can give rise to five behaviours, which can be appropriate or inappropriate (as shown in Figure 2) depending on the circumstances (Iles, 1997). Recognising the type of behaviour you prefer in a conflict situation is the first step towards a successful negotiation.

If it is impossible to get the other party to negotiate it may be necessary to withdraw, for example when a patient/client insists on a treatment that you believe is inappropriate to their clinical condition. It can be important to find ways of resisting unreasonable demands while at the same time avoiding resentment.

Reflection

For many, informal negotiating is a part of everyday working life. When working in a team you may, for example, suggest the order in which everyone will go to meal breaks on that shift to the other team members. If someone does not like the suggestions they will usually offer an alternative. Other examples of negotiations in which you may have been involved recently might include:

- a member of staff wants to change their hours or have a day off;
- staff want to increase the budget;
- staff want to decrease their workload;
- a change of staff working hours.

It is normally easy to come to a compromise and few members of staff will consider the conversation as a negotiation or a conflict.

1. Think of the times at work when you negotiated in an everyday situation such as those listed above.
2. Using Figure 2, reflect on how you normally deal with a negotiating situation. (See Negotiation.)

Stages in negotiations

Stage 1: preparation

When preparing for a negotiation you need to consider:

1. The people involved. What do you know about them? What do you think their concerns and motivations are? What do you think they want from this negotiation? While what you assume may not be correct, it can give you a framework from which to work. You can confirm their

concerns with them and you can reflect on what you could offer that might address their concerns.

2. Your objectives. Your priorities should be clear. What is your bottom line? You also need to decide what can be traded and what concessions you can make.
3. The structure of the negotiation. What has to be done in which order? The negotiation should follow a logical sequence so that details are not forgotten.
4. Your behaviour. Is the type of behaviour you normally use in a negotiating situation appropriate in a work situation? If not, how are you going to ensure that your behaviour is suitable?

Stage 2: the conduct of the process

Next, you need to decide how you will conduct the negotiation. Consider the following points:

- Before starting you should decide your tactics.
- Try to anticipate all the variables that could be on the negotiating table.
- Do you have the power of reward, even if this just involves an agreement.
- Can you use a threat of punishment – for example, not to provide an agreement
- Aim high – you can always lower your sights.

It is a human tendency to want to win when negotiating but, if the management always plays to win, you could increase conflict within the organisation. This is because, if the management always wins and the workforce always loses, this can lead to feelings of hopelessness and apathy.

Reflection

If you have ever bought a house, reflect on the process. Most people set out with an ideal house in mind, such as an old country cottage with roses round the door and a lovely garden. What they end up with is a terraced house on a main road in an estate with a small yard that has optimistically been called a garden by the estate agent. Your bottom line was the need to have a house. There were few cottages and they were out of your price range. The garden is a compromise; you can always put the work in later.

1. Think of a recent situation in which you negotiated an outcome. Did you decide where you would compromise beforehand or did you end up compromising during the negotiation when you had little choice?

Your interpersonal behaviour in the negotiation can make a lot of difference to the outcome. You are more likely to have a favourable outcome if you have some rapport with, and demonstrate respect for, the other side. The stance you take may be influenced by previous negotiations with the same person/people. If these negotiations had a successful outcome then it is worth referring back to identify your critical success factors.

You should show a willingness to come to a conclusion, but you must keep the whole package in mind, even while searching for variables that may or may not be traded. Concessions (implied or otherwise) that cost little can be traded and, when concessions are given by you, you should optimise them while minimising any concession you receive in return.

Negotiating techniques

Here are some useful negotiating techniques.

- Start with a neutral subject – in British culture it is polite to start off on a neutral subject (such as the weather). Other cultures have different customs.
- It is useful to state repeatedly the value of what you are offering.
- Present a clear explanation, summarise frequently and keep notes.
- Constraints and variables are often interchangeable.
- Ask questions to clarify points.
- Use silence.
- Read between the lines. What do they really want? Listen to what the other side are really saying and be aware of their non-verbal language.
- Sometimes it is easier to negotiate with more than one person on your side (as in interviewing). It can also help to exchange notes privately at intervals.
- Do not get hung up on deadlines – keep thinking.
- Maintain neutrality and objectivity.
- Do not make a final offer until everything is on the table.
- Leave the other party feeling good.

(Forsyth, 1991)

Some final thoughts on negotiation

A willingness and ability to negotiate is essential for a flexible and happy working environment. It is very much an interactive activity. There are two sides to all negotiations and the workforce must be prepared to negotiate, but the climate in which negotiations take place is a management responsibility. Refusal to negotiate leads to conflict. A culture of give and take where all persons are treated with respect and everyone has the right to have an opinion will reduce conflict. Creating such a culture is within most managers' remit.

The manager as arbitrator

Situations can arise, which did not involve you as manager, where arbitration is required between individuals and/or parties, such as for example, direct conflict between two members of staff. In such a situation the role of the manager is to resolve the conflict in the interests of a harmonious working atmosphere. The manager should help the parties involved find a resolution that allows them to make realistic decisions and move forward. In such situations the manager should be objective, not allowing personal feelings or relationships to influence decision making.

Adhering to set policies and procedures can help the manager avoid bias and provide a basis for dealing fairly with a situation. In the past, moving staff to other areas was used as a way to alleviate a situation. It is now considered more effective in the long term to attempt to understand the causes of the conflict and resolve them. The manager can act as a catalyst to encourage both parties involved to reflect on their roles in the situation and to help them develop strategies to overcome the difficulties. Some conflicts can escalate over a period of time so the manager needs to be observant for signs of potential breakdown in relationships. Such signs may include:

- Changes in atmosphere within a ward or unit.
- Non-specific complaints about an individual's attitude or behaviour.
- An increase in absence when individuals are allocated to work together.

Challenging behaviour can be difficult but when warning signs are ignored, a total breakdown in relationships may occur involving other staff and having consequences for patient care. Further information on arbitration can be found at **www.acas.org.uk/index.aspx?articleid=336**.

Key Learning Points

Negotiators need to understand:

- The complex processes involved;
- The stages of negotiation;
- How to conduct negotiations;
- The role of the manager as arbitrator.

DEALING WITH COMPLAINTS

If the culture of an organisation is such that all persons are treated with respect, dealing with complaints should be straightforward. Each organisation should have a procedure for dealing with complaints and all staff should be made aware of this procedure. Good complaints procedures are reliant on staff communication skills and have the following factors in common:

- Complaints should be received graciously:
  o it is important to realise that few complaints are personal, though a complaint can feel like a personal attack;
  o while you may not agree with the complaint, it is the complainant's point of view and must be treated with respect;
  o few complainants intend harm.
- All complaints should be dealt with in a timely fashion and a standard should be set for the time taken to address complaints (see Chapter 12: Information and Quality Management).
- A time limit should be set for sending a written acknowledgement of a complaint, for example within five working days of receiving the complaint.
- There should also be a reasonable time limit set for investigating the complaint (for example, 21 working days) and for sending a reply to the complainant stating the result of the investigations (for example, within 28 working days).
- The complainant should also be given the opportunity to meet with a representative of the organisation if it is felt that the complaint has not been resolved satisfactorily.
- It is important to apologise if there have been failings on the part of the organisation, and to outline the attempts that have been made to rectify matters.

A system for internal complaints should also be set up so that it is easy for patients and relatives to complain. Complaints should be viewed as a means of improving the quality of care given.

Reflection

According to their publicity, a reputable national chain store always prided itself on listening to complaints. In practice, in our local store of three floors, it was very difficult to make a complaint. At the pay point a complainant was directed to pick up a complaints form on the next floor as only one pay point in the store held forms. If you took the trouble to find and fill in the form and to send it, you did get a letter, but the store never acknowledged they were at fault. For example, if you said you could not find a certain popular size in white underwear, the letter would tell you that the sizes available in the store were calculated scientifically, and if you were having trouble it would be sensible to travel 40 miles to a larger store. Most people would be even more sensible and go to the adjacent chain store. Needless to say, the store had financial problems during this period.

1. Do you encourage patients or relatives to make comments on the care given? How do you encourage them? (See Dealing with Complaints.)

Within the organisation, staff should be encouraged to view complaints positively as a means of illustrating how the service is seen by their clients.

- Complaints should be monitored, recorded, collated and analysed.
- Staff should be actively involved in using complaints to improve their service and rectify deficiencies.

It is also vital to ensure that any letters of praise received are also passed on to staff, as there is a tendency to emphasise poor performance without acknowledging good care. It is important to remember that if mistakes occur, staff managers should be objective and non-judgemental. Staff should be given the opportunity to explain their side of events and staff should be treated with respect when you are dealing with complaints.

Reflection

When I was working in A&E many complaints were received. Despite all our efforts to forestall them, delays at busy times were inevitable. When a complaint was received one manager would ask the member of staff concerned for their explanation of the incident and if there had been poor practice, it was discussed privately. Another manager would treat every complaint as the result of poor practice and was aggressive with the members of staff concerned until it had been proved otherwise. Only one manager was respected by the staff and any comments made were taken seriously.

1. How do you deal with any staff concerned in a complaint? Are your staff involved in the analysis of complaints? Do you encourage suggestions for ways in which deficiencies can be rectified? (See Dealing with Complaints.)

Key Learning Points

Dealing with complaints requires:

- Courtesy and understanding;
- A structured process with stages and time limits;
- Objectivity and analysis rather than automatic 'blaming'.

Summary of Key Learning Points

When dealing with conflict it is important to understand:

- The sources of conflict;
- The sources of power within the organisation;
- The management of confrontations.

Negotiators need to understand:

- The complex processes involved;
- The stages of negotiation;
- How to conduct negotiations;
- The role of the manager as arbitrator.

Dealing with complaints requires:

- Courtesy and understanding;
- A structured process with stages and time limits;
- Objectivity and analysis rather than automatic 'blaming'.

Case study 1

You would like to change the times of patients' meals. At present, the last meal of the day is at 5 p.m. and the next is breakfast at 8 a.m. These times have evolved to ensure that kitchen staff will not have to work overtime. You would also like to ensure that, if patients would like larger portions, they will be available.

1. How would you set about the negotiation with the kitchen staff?
2. What information do you require?
3. What compromises can you make?

Case study 2

Mr Howlett is the manager of a home that is part of a smaller chain with a reputation locally for providing good terms and conditions for its employees. Staff, residents and relatives are all happy with the quality of care and the personal touch that the home offers. However, the reality is that in an increasingly competitive world it is becoming harder for the company, with its core values but smaller infrastructure, to remain financially viable.

The company has agreed a takeover with a larger company and the information has reached the home. The manager has his own concerns about the takeover, the future direction of the home and potential changes that are likely as a result. There is anger from the majority of people within the home and the manager is concerned that this is going to have a detrimental effect on the general atmosphere and the quality of life of the residents. He therefore finds himself in a situation where he needs to put aside his own concern and act as an objective negotiator.

1. What can the manager do to help the staff and himself come to terms with the situation?

Activities

1. Reflect on how you normally deal with negotiations in a social setting. Does this differ from how you negotiate with patients/clients and colleagues?
2. How would you deal with a patient/client who insists on an inappropriate treatment?
3. Examine your complaints procedure. Does it have time limits? Do you keep to the time limits?

Chapter 15

Introduction to models of strategic planning

INTRODUCTION

The topic of models of strategic planning will enable you to address National Occupational Standards A4 'Contribute to improvements at work' and SNH4U1 'Develop programmes, projects and plans'. In this chapter you will:

- consider models of strategic planning and change;
- gain an understanding of the principles of strategic decision making;
- examine models of strategic change;
- learn how to implement effective strategies and plans;
- gain an understanding of organisational structures and processes;
- learn how to evaluate strategies;
- gain an understanding of the influence of National Standards Frameworks on strategic planning for health and social care.

STRATEGIC PLANNING

There is no single definition of strategy, but most managers would agree with Mintzberg and Quinn that strategy is a:

> Pattern or plan that integrates an organisation's major goals, policies and action sequences into a cohesive whole.
>
> (Mintzberg and Quinn, 1991, p. 5)

The concept of strategy was first used by the Macedonian King Phillip and his son Alexander the Great in the formation of a military plan that was used to overcome their enemies and aid their conquest of other lands.

A strategy should consist of (see Figure 1):

- Goal/s   Which state what and when but not how.
- Objectives   Give overall direction and viability – strategic goals.
- Policies   Rules or guidelines within which action should occur.
- Programmes   A step-by-step sequence necessary to achieve objectives.

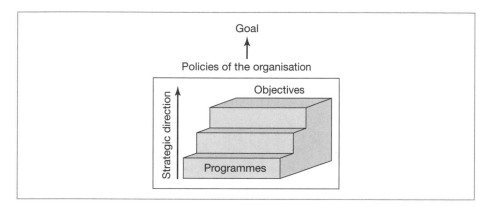

Figure 1 Strategic planning

Strategic decisions determine the overall direction of an enterprise over a period of time, during which both predicted and unpredicted changes can occur in the environment. Strategic decisions should be relevant and flexible and able to withstand the unknowable.

Reflection

In chess each player has a goal, which is to win the game. There are rules guiding the movements of each piece. A castle can only move horizontally or vertically, a bishop can only move diagonally on either black or white squares. Players must adhere to the rules (policies). There are sequences (programmes) which, when played, may achieve the goal. Before each move a successful player should work out the likely consequences of their chosen action. Opponents may, of course, produce unexpected moves that then have to be taken into consideration. Chess is an excellent game for teaching strategic thinking.

1. Does your organisation have an overall strategic goal? What is it?

MODELS OF STRATEGIC CHANGE

Mintzberg and Quinn (1991) suggest that there are different patterns and models of strategic change, ranging from deliberate strategy at one end of the scale to emergent strategy at the other end (see Figure 2). The formation of strategy is not an even process. It is dependent on the outside influences at the time and the organisational culture itself. In health and social care the influences are varied but all organisations, from the National Health Service to a small care home, exist within a framework of legislation and standards that create the deliberate strategy. Emergent strategies will be shaped by local conditions. Care homes can be owned by large national charities or businesses or may be small local businesses owned by individuals so approaches to strategic change may be very varied and exist on any part of the continuum from deliberate to emergent. Frequent changes in legislation may lead to continual changes in strategies.

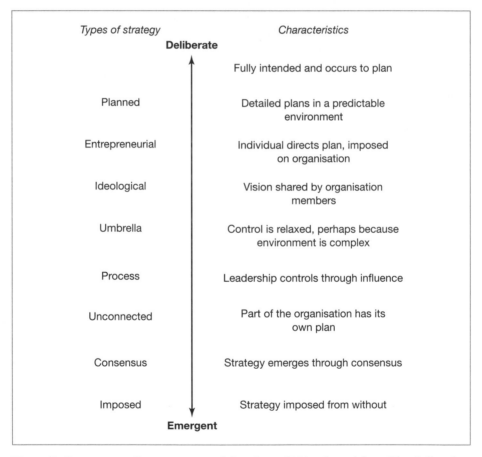

Figure 2 Continuum of strategic types (Mintzberg, 1991, adapted from Blundell and Murdoch, 1997, p. 202)

Deliberate strategy

Deliberate strategy is defined by three conditions:

1. A definite organisational intention to outline the strategy.
2. All members of the organisation should share the strategic intention.
3. Events have gone as planned.

(Blundell and Murdoch, 1997)

Emergent strategy

Emergent strategy arises when consequences, which had not been intended by the actions taken, evolve. Consequences can arise from an immediate response to a situation and as such the effects may be unforeseen.

> ### Reflection
>
> Farmers in the European Union were producing surpluses of crops. It was decided to pay them to 'set aside' land, which should, in theory, reduce crop surpluses. In fact, the surpluses remained because farmers 'set aside' their least productive land and bought fertiliser with the money they received, with the result that their crop yields increased on the land in production.
>
> 1. The situation above is the 'law of unintended consequences'. Can you think of similar situations in health and social care services? (See Strategic Planning.)

Strategic levels

There are strategies at different management levels in an organisation and these should form a cohesive whole. For example, a ward (operational) strategy should be consistent with a departmental (business level) strategy, which should in turn be part of a coherent corporate strategy. The large charities and businesses that run multiple homes will set the corporate strategy and the homes should implement operational strategies that will enable them to meet the corporation's overall goals and programmes. Strategic decisions have major resource implications affecting the operation of an organisation over a period of time, so it is vital that strategies at all levels of an organisation are fully integrated into the overall corporate strategy.

EFFECTIVE STRATEGIES

To be effective it is essential that the most important strategic goals should be achieved within the framework of guiding policies which limit the action that can be taken. The defined goals should be achieved through defined programmes. The key concepts of effective strategy are that it is:

- cohesive;
- balanced;
- focused;
- resourced;
- and controlled.

Effective strategies must also:

- deal with the predictable and unpredictable;
- have flexibility built in;
- affect the organisation over a period of time;
- have clear objectives;
- be co-ordinated throughout the organisation.

Complex organisations should have a number of hierarchically related and mutually supportive strategies. Many organisations use a 'mission statement' to help clarify the organisation's purpose, values and behaviour.

Reflection

Organisations are expected to have a strategic direction that is summed up in a mission statement that is clear and that every person in the organisation understands. A visitor to British Airways asked a cleaner what was the main objective of the organisation. 'To keep the planes flying' came back the answer.

1. Does your organisation have a mission statement? Does it reflect the main purpose of the organisation? (See Effective Strategies.)

Key Learning Points

Strategic planning requires:

- Goals, policies and programmes;
- Awareness of unintended consequences;
- Awareness that different levels of the business have different plans;
- That effective strategies must be cohesive, balanced, focused, resourced and controlled.

STRATEGIES AND PLANS

> Strategy is a unified, comprehensive and integrated plan ... designed to ensure that the basic objectives of the enterprise are achieved.
>
> (Gleuck, 1980)

Strategies that remain in the mind of the manager are never going to benefit the organisation. To be effective they must be shared in the organisation, with everyone committed to the strategy and playing their part. Newcomers to the organisation should have an induction that includes the mission statement and the overall plans and goals of the organisation. Changes in goals and plans must be communicated to the whole organisation. Corporate strategy is reflected in the pattern of decisions in a company, which includes its:

- goals;
- policies;
- plans;
- range of business;
- human relations;
- selection of strategic criteria.

Organisations need to ensure that their strategic plan:

- meets its aims and objectives;
- builds on its strengths and attempts to overcome its weaknesses;
- enables it to seize opportunities and counter threats.

Organisational processes

The way in which a strategy is put into action is inseparable from the structure, behaviour and culture of the company in which it has been developed. In a bureaucracy strategies will be formal and their implementation will be organised via job descriptions and roles. In a team or task-oriented culture strategies will be implemented by the team based on expertise (Handy, 1999). Resources should be available to enable the organisation to achieve the strategy.

Strategic implementation

The strengths and weaknesses of the organisation should be analysed and it is important not to lose sight of the core business. In the social care sector the core business can be very varied and will range from rehabilitation to end of life care. Making a profit may also be core business if it is imperative for the business to survive.

> ## Reflection
>
> It is relatively easy for a firm that produces one type of product to understand its core business. In health and care services it can be a disadvantage to concentrate only on the core business. In the mid-1980s, the government encouraged hospitals and health care institutions to sell off their residential property. The government argued that their core business was health care, not renting property. However, as property prices rose in the cities, the institutions that had sold their property had difficulty in recruiting staff, as market rents and house prices rose beyond the reach of most essential workers.
>
> 1. What supports your core business and enables it to survive? (See Strategic implementation.)

In order to implement a strategy it is essential to ensure that you have the following in place first:

- resources;
- staff;
- finance;
- information;
- operational capability (that may mean training staff).

(Blundell and Murdoch, 1997)

Organisational structures and processes

When you are drawing up plans based on your strategy you need to ensure the structures of your organisation are appropriate and are able to co-ordinate the planned activities. For example, if you are going to use a team structure the teams must be appropriately led and members must understand their responsibilities. Similarly, organisational processes must result in behaviour that achieves the organisation's purpose and is appropriate for the structure. Teams work best in organisations that are good at communications and have flat (non-hierarchical) structures that encourage everyone to be part of the team. This has created problems in the health service where ward teams and multidisciplinary teams try to work in a hierarchical structure where they are expected to work to their job descriptions, which causes difficulties with role boundaries and affects the way the team works. (See Chapter 5: Team Building.)

Leadership

Leadership is vital when you are implementing strategy. Strong leadership can help compensate for organisational weaknesses. (See Chapter 4: Leadership.)

Reflection

To achieve your strategic goals it is important to have an effective leader. Think of the effective generals in history such as Napoleon, the Duke of Wellington and, in the Second World War, General Montgomery. All were single-minded and they ensured that they had an organisation that was fit for purpose, which was to win. The Trusts that have been successful in the health service have had good leadership, as have successful national and international corporations and political parties.

1. Have you ever worked in an organisation that was effective in achieving its strategic goals? If so, what part did the leader play?

Risk-taking

Strategic planning involves some risk-taking as nothing is certain in the future. It is, however, possible to estimate the actual or the potential capacity of an organisation to take advantage of the likely market needs and its ability to cope with any risks that this involves.

Reflection

With the numbers of elderly increasing in the population, there was an assumption that the market for residential homes would increase. Many of the clients were funded by social services when they were unable to pay. However, the government introduced new legislation, the NHS and Community Care Act, in 1990 that stated that patients had to be assessed prior to admission and the emphasis switched to giving assistance to the elderly to enable them to stay in their own homes. Many residential home owners who had overextended their financial commitments were forced to close.

1. You should be aware of any national legislation that affects you or is likely to affect you in the future. Is there anything in the government's current legislative programme that could have a similar effect to the 1990 Act?

Alternative strategies should be examined and the level of risk that the organisation can accept should be kept in mind when the opportunities are analysed. The level to which a company can accept risk will depend on what a company produces.

> ## Reflection
>
> In health and social care it is imperative to avoid as much risk as possible as it may have severe consequences for the patient. There are moves to encourage the patient to actively participate in accepting a level of risk, such as for example, with the issue of informed consent. In this case, it can be difficult for patients to estimate the risks of, for example, taking an antibiotic that they have never taken before. You know the antibiotic can have side effects, but you don't know if you will be affected and you may not have any side effects. Similarly we accept that we may not reach the other side every time we cross a road, so it is a risk we take and accept.
>
> 1. How does your organisation manage risk? (See Risk taking.)

Strategy is often a compromise between the following factors. Organisations need to decide:

What they might do	*v*	What they want to do
What they can do	*v*	What they should do

THE EVALUATION OF STRATEGIES

There is a need to have a formal and consistent system for evaluating your strategy. A strategy must adapt to changes in the external environment. Companies work in an environment that is constantly changing; technology advances, economic factors alter, as do physical, social and political expectations. It is essential to continually monitor the environment, to ensure that strategies remain relevant and feasible (see Figure 3). An acronym which can be used to analyse the environment is PESTeL, the letters of which stand for:

- Political factors;
- Economic factors;
- Social factors;
- Technical factors;
- Legal factors.

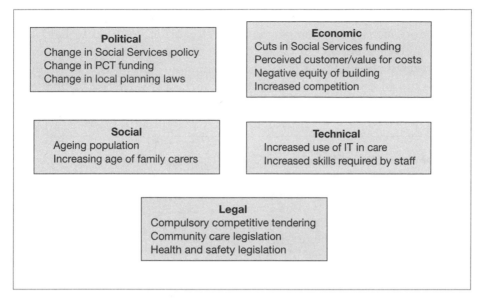

Figure 3 A PESTeL analysis for a care home (adapted from Blundell and Murdoch,1997, p. 211)

Strategic planning is essentially an analytical process, which must be continually monitored to detect any discontinuity with the planned strategy (see Figure 4). It is important to know the business and its history, to understand any patterns of change or continuity that will need to be reconciled to the strategic goal. Stability needs to be managed and change should only be undertaken when it is necessary.

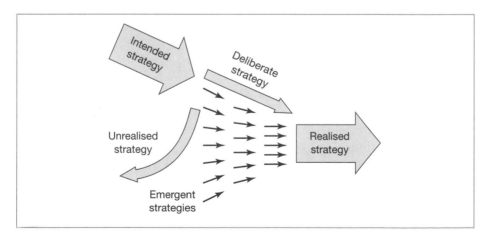

Figure 4 Deliberate and emergent strategies

Strategy is imposed as a top-down goal with a rational and formal outcome, but it should also be seen as a continuous process. It will evolve as it is influenced by previous decisions, emergent strategies and policy. In health and social care strategic planning it is often destined to failure as there is no single product or range of products that allows rationalisation in the interests of efficiency. Consumer behaviour can also be difficult to understand in the context of health and social care. There can be a tendency to deal with present problems but not to plan for the future.

Key Learning Points

Within organisations strategic planning depends on:

- The structure and policies of the organisation;
- The leadership of the organisation;
- The organisation's attitude to risk;
- The organisation's approach to management.

NATIONAL STANDARDS FRAMEWORKS

The introduction of National Standards Frameworks is a deliberate attempt by the government to address the difficulties of strategic planning in health and social care. The new guidelines set out a:

> Standard-based planning framework for health and social care and standards for NHS health care to be used in planning, commissioning and delivering services.
>
> (Department of Health, 2004, p. 1)

Sir Nigel Crisp describes the framework's purpose as:

> ... an integrated approach which brings together for the first time the planning framework, national standards and the new Payment by Results system to provide a clear direction of travel and incentives for local organisations.
>
> (Department of Health, 2004, p. 3)

Social care services are responsible for implementing the framework, with a focus on health and wellbeing across the whole system. Health organisations and Local Authorities are required to work closer together across the range of health and social care services, within a partnership framework of local targets.

Social care sector strategic planning will also be affected by the Department of Health's (2004) drive to give users of their services more power to improve their care by directing the system. Particular attention will be paid to clients with long-term conditions, the promotion of independence for older people, the support of self-care and the 'expert patient' (Department of Health, 2004, p.5).

The National Standards will be implemented in relation to National Service Frameworks, and the Commission for Social Care Inspection (CSCI) will be responsible for ensuring compliance within the social care sector. The emphasis will be placed on supporting people in their own homes and preventing admission to either hospital or the long-term care sector (Department of Health, 2004).

Key Learning Points

Strategic planning is affected by:

- National Standards Frameworks;
- The emphasis on supporting people in their own homes;
- Changing patterns in the allocation of resources, including payment by results.

Summary of Key Learning Points

Strategic planning requires:

- Goals, policies and programmes;
- Awareness of unintended consequences;
- Awareness that different levels of the business have different plans;
- That effective strategies must be cohesive, balanced, focused, resourced and controlled.

Within organisations strategic planning depends on:

- The structure and policies of the organisation;
- The leadership of the organisation;
- The organisation's attitude to risk;
- The organisation's approach to management.

Strategic planning is affected by:

- National Standards Frameworks;
- The emphasis on supporting people in their own homes;
- Changing patterns in the allocation of resources, including payment by results.

Activities

1. Have you evolved your own strategic plan for your life? For example, have you planned how you can manage to buy a house? What factors did you take into account?
2. Analyse the strategic plan for your organisation. Does it appear to meet the aims and objectives of the organisation and build on its strengths? Will it enable the organisation to take advantage of any economic opportunities? (See Figure 1 on page 213.)
3. Try evaluating the environment in which your organisation works. What aspects of the environment could affect your organisation? (See Figure 3 on page 221.)
4. How will the National Standards Frameworks affect strategic planning in your organisation?

Case study 1

You are a manager in a residential home and the owners, a large organisation, have decided to enlarge the home to include some nursing home beds. They have also decided to admit clients with Alzheimer disease to both parts of the home and plan that the new beds will be open in 18 months. As a manager you will be responsible for writing a strategic plan to ensure that you have the appropriate expertise among your staff to care for all the patients.

1. What knowledge and expertise do you need to do this?

Case study 2

You would like to become a care home manager. At present you are working in a small care home and the owner is the manager and there is also an assistant manager in the home, neither of whom is likely to leave their jobs in the next five years. You live in a large town and there are other care homes in the town.

1. How are you going to strategically plan your career?

References

BOOKS AND JOURNAL ARTICLES

Adair, J. (1973) *Action-Centred Leadership*. Gower

Adair, J. (1987) *Effective Teambuilding*. Pan Macmillan

Adair, J. (ed.) (1999) *Adair on Leadership*. Hawksmere, Neil Thomas

Bailey, D. (1998) *NHS Budget Holder's Survival Guide*. Royal Society of Medicine Press Ltd

Banner, D.K. and Cooke, R.A. (1984) 'Ethical dilemmas in performance appraisal'. *Journal of Business Ethics*, 3, 4 November, pp. 327–33

Beardwell, I., Holden, L. and Clydon, T. (eds) (2004) *Human Resource Management: A Contemporary Approach* 4th edn. Financial Times, Prentice Hall

Belbin, R.M. (1993) *Team Roles at Work: A Strategy for Human Resource Management*. Butterworth-Heinemann

Benner, P. (1984) *From Novice to Expert*. Addison Wesley Publishing Company

Blundell, B. and Murdoch, A., (1997) *Managing in the Public Sector*. Butterworth-Heinemann

Bolton, L.B., Jones, D., Aydin, C.E., Donaldson, N., Brown, D.S., Lowe, M., McFarland, P.L. and Harms, D. (2001) 'A response to California's mandated nurse ratios'. *Journal of Nursing Scholarship*, 33:2, pp. 179–84

Boud, D., Keogh, R. and Walker, D. (1988) *Reflection: Turning Experience into Learning*. Kogan Page

Broody, R. (2005) *Effectively Managing Human Service Organizations* 3rd edn. Sage Publications

Bryans, W. (2005) *Resource Management in Health and Social Care, Essential Checklists*. Radcliffe Publishing

Buchanan, D. and Boddy, D. (1992) *The Expertise of the Change Agent*. Prentice Hall

Buchanan, D. and Huczynski, A. (2004) *Organizational Behaviour* 5th edn. Prentice Hall

Buchan, J. and Seccombe, I. (2003) *More nurses, working differently? A review of the UK nursing labour market 2002–2003*. Review prepared by Queen Margaret University College, Edinburgh and published by the Royal College of Nursing, London

Buerhaus, P.I., Staiger, D.O. and Auerbach, D.I. (2000) 'Implications of an ageing Registered Nurse workforce'. *Journal of the American Medical Association*, 283:22, 14 June, pp. 2948–54

Calnan, M. (1987) *Health & Illness: The Lay Perspective.* Tavistock Publications

Carr-Hill, R., Dixon, P.G. and Gibbs, L. (1992) *Skill Mix and the Effectiveness of Nursing Care.* Centre for Health Care Economics, University of York

Cohen, L., Manion, L. and Morrison, K. (2000) *Research Methods in Education* 5th edn. Routledge

Cole, G.A. (1990) *Management Theory and Practice.* D.P. Publications Ltd

Cole G.A. (1997) *Personnel Management: Theory and Practice.* D.P. Publications Ltd

Cole, G.A. (2002) *Personnel and Human Resource Management* 5th edn. Continuum

Crossan, F. and Ferguson, D. (2005) 'Exploring nursing skill mix: a review'. *Journal of Nursing Management*, 13, pp. 356–62

Currie, D. (2006) *Introduction to Human Resource Management: A Guide to Personnel in Practice.* Chartered Institute of Personnel and Development

Currie, V., Harvey, G., West, E., McKenna, H. and Keeney, S. (2005) 'Relationship between quality of care, staffing levels, skill mix and nurse autonomy: literature review'. *Journal of Advanced Nursing*, 51:1, pp. 73–82

Department of Health (1993) *A Vision for the Future.* HMSO

Department of Health (1997a) *The Caldicott Committee Report on the Review of Patient-Identifiable Information.* Department of Health

Department of Health (1997b) *Implementing the Caldicott Standard into Social Care.* Department of Health

Department of Health (2000) *No Secrets.* Department of Health and Home Office

Department of Health (2001) *Making a Difference.* Department of Health

Department of Health (2002) *Implementing the Caldicott Standard into Social Care.* Local Authority circular. Crown copyright

Department of Health (2003) *Care Homes for Older People. National Minimum Standards.* Crown Copyright

Department of Health (2004) *National Standards, Local Action: Health and Social Care Standards and Planning Framework 2005/06–2007/08.* Department of Health.

Department of Health (2007) *National Electronic Social Care Record Survey Report – 2006/07.* Department of Health

Dewey, J. (1933) *How We Think* revised edn. D.C. Heath and Co.

Donaldson, L. (1995) 'Management for Doctors: conflict, power, negotiation'. *British Medical Journal*, 310:104–7

Dopson, S. and Stewart, R. (1993) 'Information technology, organizational restructuring and the future of middle management'. *New Technology Work and Employment*, 8:1 pp10–20

Driscoll, J. (2000) *Practising Clinical Supervision: A Reflective Approach.* Bailliere Tindall

Etzioni, A. (1964) *Modern Organisations.* Prentice Hall Inc.

Feuer, L. (2003) 'The management challenge: making the most of your next performance appraisal'. *Total Quality Management*, Sept/Oct, pp. 22–4

Fiedler, F.E. (1967) *A Theory of Leadership Effectiveness.* McGraw-Hill

Flanagan, H. and Spurgeon, P. (1996) *Public Sector Managerial Effectiveness.* Open University Press

Fondas, N. and Stewart, R. (1994) 'Enactment in managerial jobs: A role analysis'. *Journal of Management Studies* 31:1 Jan pp. 83–103.

Forsyth, P. (1991) *How to Negotiate Successfully*. Sheldon Press

Fowler, A. (1996) *Negotiation: Skills and Strategies*. Institute of Personnel Management

Gleuck, W.F. and Juach, L.R. (1980) *Strategic Management and Business Policy* 2nd edn. Addison-Wesley

Gould, T. and Merrett, H. (1992) *Introducing Quality Assurance in the NHS*. Macmillan

Guba, E.J. and Lincoln, Y.S. (1985) *Naturalistic Inquiry*. In Cohen, L., Manion, L. and Morrison, K. (2000) *Research Methods in Education* 5th edn. Routledge

Hales, C. P. (1986) 'What do managers do? A critical review of the evidence'. *Journal of Management Studies* 23:1 pp. 88–115

Handy, C.B. (1986) *Gods of Management* 3rd edn. Century Business

Handy, C.B. (1999) *Understanding Organizations* 4th edn. Penguin Books

Hannagan, T. (1998) *Management Concepts and Pratices* 2nd edn. Pitman Publishing

Hardy, J. (2005) 'Students are well-placed to be interdepartmental peacekeepers'. *Nursing Standard*, 20:4, p. 72

Harrington, H.J. (1998) 'Perspective performance improvement: Was W. Edwards Deming wrong?'. *The TQM Magazine*, 10, 4, pp. 230–7

Huczynski, A. and Buchanan, D. (1991) *Organizational Behaviour* 2nd edn. Prentice Hall Inc.

Huczynski, A. and Buchanan, D. (2001) *Organizational Behaviour* 4th edn. Prentice Hall Inc.

Huczynski, A. and Buchanan, D. (2004) *Organizational Behaviour* 4th edn. Prentice Hall Inc.

Hunt, J.W. (1992) *Managing People at Work*. McGraw-Hill

Hunter, D.J. (1995) 'Creating health services strategy'. In Glynn, J.J. and Perkins, D.A., (1995) *Managing Health Care*. W.B. Saunders Co. Ltd

Hurst, K. (2002) *Selecting and Applying Methods for Estimating the Size and Mix of Nursing Teams*. Nuffield Institute for Health

Iles, V. (1997) *Really Managing Health Care*. Open University Press

Information Commissioner's Office (2007) *Data Protection Act and the Freedom of Information Act*. Information Commissioner's Office

Jasper, M. (2003) *Beginning Reflective Practice*. Nelson Thornes Ltd

Johns, C. (1995) 'Achieving effective work as a professional activity'. In Schober, J.E. and Hinchliff, S.M. (1992) (eds) *Towards Advanced Practice: Key Concepts for Health Care*, pp 252–80. Arnold

Jones, A. and McDonnell, U. (1993) *Managing the Clinical Resource*. Bailliere Tindall

Juran Institute (1993) *Quality Improvement – Health Care Team Preparation Workbook*. Juran Institute

Katz, D. and Kahn, R.L. (1978) *The Social Psychology of Organizations* 2nd edn. John Wiley and Sons Ltd

Kogan, M. and Redfern, S. (1995) *Making Use of Clinical Audit: A Guide to Practice in the Health Professions*. Open University

Kolb, D. (1984) *Experiential Learning as the Science of Learning and Development.* Prentice Hall

Kovner, C., Mezey, M. and Harrington, C. (2000) 'Research priorities for staffing, case mix and quality of care in US nursing homes'. *Journal of Nursing Scholarship,* 33:1, pp. 77–80

Lee, T.-Y., Yeh M.-L., Chen, H.-H. and Lien, G.-H. (2005) 'The skill mix practice model for nursing: measuring outcome'. *Journal of Advanced Nursing,* 51:4, pp. 406–13

Lewin, K. (1951) *Field Theory in Social Science.* Harper and Row

Lewin, K., Lippitt, R. and White, R.K. (1939) 'Patterns of aggressive behaviour in experimentally created social climates'. *Journal of Social Psychology,* 10, 271–9 **[http://faculty.css.edu/dswenson/web/LEAD/lippit&white.html]**

Likert, R. (1961) *New Patterns of Management.* McGraw-Hill

Lippitt, G.L. (1973) *Visualising Change, Model Building and the Change Process.* University Associates Inc.

Lord Laming (2003) *The Victoria Climbié Inquiry.* Home Office

Madzar, S. (1997) 'Perspective hungry for feedback?'. *Management Development Review,* 10:6/7, pp. 246–8

Martin, V. and Henderson, E. (2001) *Managing in Health and Social Care.* Routledge

Mintzberg, H. (1983) *Power in and Around Organizations.* Prentice Hall Inc.

Mintzberg, H. and Quinn, J.B. (1991) *The Strategy Process.* Prentice Hall Inc.

McGregor, D. (1960) *The Human Side of Enterprise.* McGraw-Hill

National Health Service and Community Care Act 1990. Office of Public Sector Information

NHS Management Executive (1993) *A vision for the future: the Nursing, Midwifery and health visiting contribution to care.* Department of Health.

Palmer, A., Burns, S. and Bulman, C. (eds) (1994) *Reflective Practice in Nursing: The Growth of the Professional Practitioner.* Blackwell Scientific Publications

Pearson, A. (1998) 'Quantity or quality – developing a nursing workforce for the future'. Editorial in *International Journal of Nursing Practice,* 4, pp. 205

Pettigrew, H., Ferlie, E. and McKee, L. (1992) *Shaping Strategic Change.* Sage Publications

Plant, R. (1995) *Managing Change and Making it Stick.* HarperCollins

Pronovost, P.J., Dang, D., Dorman, T., Lipsett, P.A., Garrett, E., Jenckes, M. and Bass, E.P. (2001) 'Intensive care unit nurse staffing and the risk for complications after abdominal aortic surgery'. *Effective Clinical Practice,* 4:5, pp. 199-206

RCN (2001) *Determining safe staffing levels.* Royal College of Nursing, London

Richards, H. and Heginbotham, C. (1992) *Enquire: Quality Assurance through Observation of Service Delivery: A Workbook* 2nd edn. King's Fund

Richardson, G. (1999) 'Identifying, evaluating and implementing cost-effective skill mix'. *Journal of Nursing Management,* 7, pp. 265–70

Rowntree, D. (1981) *Statistics without Tears.* Penguin Books Ltd

Sale, D. (2000) *Quality Assurance: A pathway to excellence.* Macmillan Press Ltd

Schein, E.H (1970) *Organization Psychology* 2nd edn. Prentice Hall

Scott, C. and West, E. (2004) 'Special issue on the nursing workforce unit and quality of care'. Editorial in *Journal of Nursing Management,* 12, pp. 381–4

Sergison, M. (1999) 'Skill mix in primary care – creating a bibliography'. *Health Libraries Review*, 16, pp. 106–11

Shuldham, C.M. (2004) 'Nursing skill mix and staffing'. *Journal of Nursing Management*, 12, pp. 385–7

Skinner, B.F. (1972) *Beyond Freedom and Dignity*. Bantam Books

Steinbrook, R. (2002) 'Nursing in the crossfire'. *New England Journal of Medicine*, 346:22, 30 May, pp. 1757–66

Stewart, R. (1996) *Leading in the NHS*. Macmillan Business

Stewart, R. (1997) *Really Managing*. Butterworth Heinemann

Stubbings, E. and Scott, J. (2004) 'NHS workforce issues: Implications for future practice'. *Journal of Health Organization and Management*, 18:3, pp. 179–94

Tannenbaum, R. and Schmidt, W.H. (1958) 'How to choose a leadership pattern'. *Harvard Business Review*, 36:2, March/April, pp. 95–101

Telford, W.A. (1979) 'Determining nursing establishment levels'. *Health Service Manpower Review*, 5:4, April, pp. 11–12

Thomas, A.P. (2003) *Care Management in Practice for the Registered Manager Award*. Heinemann Education

Townsend, P., Davison, N. and Whitehead, M. (1988) *Inequalities in Health: The Black Report and the Health Divide*. Penguin Books

Tuckman, B.W. (1965) 'Development sequence in small groups'. *Psychological Bulletin*, 63, pp. 384–99

Tuckman, B.W. and Jensen, M.A.C. (1977) 'Stages of small group development revisited'. *Group and Organizational Studies*, 2, pp. 419–27

Wiese, D.S. and Buckley, M.R. (1998) 'The evolution of the performance appraisal process'. *Journal of Management History*, 4, 3, pp. 233–49

WEBSITES

Learning and Development in the Department of Health, **http://www.dh.gov.uk/Policy AndGuidance/HumanResourcesAndTraining/LearningAndPersonalDevelopment /Appraisals/AppraisalsArticle/fs/en?CONTENT_ID=4080275&chk=zoQbRx**
An interesting document setting out the advantages of appraisal for medical practitioners in the NHS.

The ACAS Website with a useful section on appraisal and many other helpful documents. **http://www.acas.org.uk/index.aspx?articleid=651**

Criminal Records Bureau (2007) **www.crb.gov.uk**

Employment Equality (Age) Regulations (2006) **www.opsi.gov.uk/si/si2006/20061031.htm#7**

Equal Opportunities Commission Recruitment and Selection Checklist (2006) **www.eoc.org.uk/PDF/recruitment_and_selection_checklist.pdf**

Social Care Institute for Excellence **www.scie.org.uk/recruitment/forms/guidance.doc**

Audit Scotland (2002) 'Planning ward nursing – legacy or design?' Prepared for the Auditor General, available 18/12/02 **www.audit-scotland.gov.uk**

Batty D. (2004) Social Care Staff: the issue explained. *Society Guardian.* Tuesday January 6, 2004. **www.societyguardian.co.uk**

General Social Care Council (2007) The Social Care Register **www.gscc.org.uk/Home**

Department of Health (2007) Information for Social Care. **www.dh.gov.uk/en/Policy andguidance/Informationpolicy/Informationforsocialcare/index.htm**

Data Protection Act (1998) and the Freedom of Information Act (2002) **www.ico.gov.uk**

Department of Health (2007) Electronic Social Care Records. **www.dh.gov.uk/en/ Policyandguidance/Informationpolicy/Informationforsocialcare/ DH_4073714 www.acas.org.uk/index.aspx?articleid=336**

Index

Added to a page number 'f' denotes a figure.

I
ideas people 66
income 153
incremental budgeting 148
indirect costs 144, 152
individual supervision 20, 23
induced change 187
informal appraisal 91
information
 analysing 172–3
 checks, in recruitment 118
 decision making
  assessing trustworthiness 41
  collecting 36–7
 qualitative 174
 quality management 175
 quantitative 175
 requirements, contracting 155
 resource management 160
 sharing 175
 sources 171–2
 storage and retrieval 170–1
 for workforce planning 127–30
 see also management information
information management 170–5
 case study 185
information technology, team working 71
innovative change 188
internal advertising 112
interview styles, appraisal 102–3
interviewing (recruitment) 118–20
 avoiding bias 120
 effective questioning 120
 information checks 118
 interview formats 118–19
 location and seating arrangements 119
 number of interviewers 119–20
intrinsic theories 51
IQ tests 118

J
job content, negotiating 7–8
job descriptions 3
job-centred recruitment 110
John's model, structured reflection 16–17, 18
journals, recruitment advertisements 112
Juran trilogy of total quality management 178f

K
key relationship mapping, proposed change 193f
Kolb's model of reflection 16

L
Laming Enquiry 20
leaders 49, 64–5
Leader's Prayer 58
leadership 48–61
 behaviour 52–5
 case studies 59–60
 characteristics 55
 continuum of styles 51–2
 definitions and theories 49–52
 development and support of 56–7
 guides 56
 Handy's Leader's Prayer 58
 problems 56
 strategy implementation 218
Leading in Empowered Organisations programme 57
learning curve 189f
learning styles 78–9
legal principles, information storage and retrieval 170–1
Lewin's change theory 24f, 188–90
Likert, Rensis 50–1
linear scales, measuring performance 95–6
Lippett's change theory 24f, 189
local market, recruitment 112

M
McGregor and leadership 50
management information, appraisal process 91
managers 49
 appraisal interview styles 102–3
 as arbitrators 207
 effective 62, 65
managers' roles 7–11
 communication 9
 control 8
 decisional 33
 leadership 8
 negotiating job content 7–8
 personality and behaviour 9
 supervision, problem-solving and expertise 8